A PSYCHIATRIC PRIMER FOR THE VETERAN'S FAMILY AND FRIENDS

BY

Alexander G. Dumas, M. D.
FELLOW OF THE AMERICAN PSYCHIATRIC ASSOCIATION

AND

Grace Keen

THE UNIVERSITY OF MINNESOTA PRESS
Minneapolis

FOREWORD

About a year ago I attended a luncheon meeting called by the director of the University of Minnesota Press. Among the others present were two Twin City psychiatrists, a psychiatric social worker from the local Veterans Administration facility, a representative of the Minneapolis Family Welfare agency, and the executive secretary of the university YMCA.

We had met to discuss a problem that was being given more and more space in newspapers and magazines: the number of American men being rejected or discharged from military service because of neuropsychiatric disabilities. The evidence seemed to show that these men were returning to civilian circles in which next to nothing was known about the nature or implications of their mental and emotional difficulties. Their families and friends were facing this problem with little more than old wives' tales about psychiatric illness to guide them.

Would a book of explanation, simply and readably written, be useful in this situation? Was there the need there seemed to be for such a book? Could the necessary scientific material be suitably presented for the nonspecialist reader? And could enough of general principles and advice be given to make the book helpful to the families and friends of returning servicemen? These were the questions the director of the Press put before us.

Since most of us were already having to deal with the problem in our daily duties, we had no doubt about the need. We were somewhat less certain that it could be met in a generalized discussion, when each case is so entirely an individual matter. But we thought it was worth trying and agreed to contribute what suggestions and assistance we could.

This *Psychiatric Primer for the Veteran's Family and Friends* is the result. Of its two authors, Dr. Alexander Dumas is a psychiatrist of some twenty years' experience, much of it in charge of the nervous and mental section of a Veterans Administration hospital, and Grace Keen is a writer experienced in the difficult task of making scientific material intelligible to the layman. In their collaboration Dr. Dumas has provided most of the information, the case histories, and their interpretation, and Mrs. Keen has arranged the material, put it in written form, and done the drawings to illustrate it. Not only have they handled the subject assigned them, but they have added a very useful presentation of the psychological problems of the physically disabled veteran. In my opinion they have produced a psychiatric guide that cannot fail to be helpful in the situation it was designed to meet.

While this book has been in preparation, a noteworthy change has come over some of the writing on the subject in newspapers and magazines. A number of persons have taken to print to deny, apparently with more emotion than information, that returning servicemen will have any psychological problems at all. These writers, quite unconsciously, are voicing a reaction that is all too familiar to psychologists and psychiatrists in the United States: Americans may glory in their physical ailments, but they reject with vehemence any suggestion that their minds or emotions are out of gear.

This attitude, however loudly or eloquently expressed, cannot change the facts. It is true that most veterans will readjust to the civilian world without psychiatric difficulty. But it is equally true that at least two million men have been rejected or discharged for neuropsychiatric disorders. And it is the best guess of experts that existing facilities and personnel can provide adequate psychiatric treatment for only five per cent of the veterans who will need it.

In the face of these facts, it is absurd to say that books like this *create* a problem. They are much-needed attempts to meet a problem that, whether we want to admit it or not, is real and troublesome to hundreds of thousands of our countrymen. I believe that this psychiatric guide for families and friends can be a valuable supplement to the personal treatment and counseling of the veterans themselves, and I am sure it will be welcomed as such by psychiatrists, family doctors, social workers in a host of agencies, personnel officers in business and industry, and any others who in the months and years ahead will be dealing with the personal aftermath of war.

STARKE R. HATHAWAY

August 1945
University of Minnesota

Acknowledgments

Many persons have contributed to the case histories, the advice, and the suggestions which we have here set down. Because of the confidential nature of the information they gave us, many of these contributors must remain anonymous, and we therefore think it best to thank them all without mention by name. They may be sure that our gratitude for their interest, time, and effort is nonetheless personally felt.

We are also much indebted to these who have read the manuscript in advance of publication: Dr. Thomas A. C. Rennie of the Payne Whitney Psychiatric Clinic of the New York Hospital; Mrs. Imogene S. Young, psychiatric social work consultant for the American Red Cross; J. Benjamin Schmoker, executive secretary of the YMCA in Minneapolis; Dr. Bertrum C. Schiele, psychiatrist, and Dr. Starke R. Hathaway, clinical psychologist, both of the University of Minnesota faculty. For their valuable criticisms and suggestions we are deeply grateful, but for any errors of omission or inclusion that may still remain we take full responsibility.

ALEXANDER DUMAS AND GRACE KEEN

CONTENTS

THEY REPRESENT ALL OF US

On the station platform of a midwestern town one sunny day in spring, five women are waiting for the train that will bring their menfolk back from the war.

The names of these women, who they are, and where they live, do not matter; nor does the name of the town, the train, or the date of its arrival. For the stories of these women and the men for whom they wait are told here, not because they are the stories of individuals, but because they represent the three big classes of returning servicemen for whose homecoming women throughout America are waiting: the uninjured, the physically hurt, and the mentally hurt.

The great majority of the women whose men return from war will, of course, be the fortunate ones like Ellen. But there will be all too many who must be prepared for changes like those that Mary, Betty, Sarah, and Edith are facing.

In telling the stories of these five women and their menfolk, the difficulties they face, the adjustments they must make, it is hoped that all major aspects of the veterans' return will be discussed. It is of course impossible to cover every possible problem, but the discussion and rules for the cases that are given should suggest proper methods and attitudes in others of the same general kind.

If he is uninjured . . .
GIVE HIM TIME

Ellen and Tom

Among the women waiting for the train that will bring their husbands and sons back to them as John Does rather than GI Joes, Ellen is the youngest. She is waiting for Tom, her husband, whom she married three years ago, just before he went overseas.

Ellen and Tom have known each other since childhood. They were brought up together in the same neighborhood and went to the same schools. They skated and studied and danced together, and they and their families all took it for granted that when Tom was established and earning enough they would get married.

The summer they graduated from high school Tom got a job driving an express truck and Ellen went to work as a stenographer. Then came the war, and at the end of the year Tom left his job to enlist in the army. Through various tests and interviews to determine his abilities and preferences, the army decided that he could best fit into their program as a mechanic, and after his basic training his special course began.

Tom liked this new work. He wanted to be a mechanic. But midway through his course came a sudden call for ground crews and he was ordered overseas. Then suddenly the future seemed less sure, the waiting for marriage less sensible. If he and Ellen postponed the step they might never be able to take it. So on his furlough home they were married and spent two joyous weeks together before he went away.

Tom's station was in England, and there he stayed throughout the war, his training as a mechanic never completed.

When Tom went overseas, Ellen stayed on with her family until after Tommy was born. Then she decided to return to her work as a stenographer. Tommy was not the problem for her that he might have been if her mother and Tom's had not been such willing and able "soldiers in a grandmothers' war."

At the office Ellen met other wives whose husbands were away. They formed a club, some of them, and exchanged ideas and plans for furnishing the houses or apartments they hoped to have when the war was over and their husbands came home. Their lives became ones of waiting, in which postmen and mailboxes played a major part. Strange cities and countries, oceans and seas, took on new meaning as "the place where Tom is," or John or Harry.

Although they did not talk about it and in the demands of the daily routine perhaps did not realize that it was so, the day when the boys would come marching home became the pivot on which their lives turned. They lived mostly in that future time, and in their dreams there were no shadows or clouds of any sort.

The difference a day makes

The sunlight, shining full on Ellen as she stands waiting on the station platform, makes the blue of her suit and hat even bluer than it had looked in her room. For months her suit and hat have been ready to wear, and for weeks past she has made a point of buying little articles, a handkerchief, a comb, earrings, to go with them.

As Ellen glances about at the other women, the thought occurs to her that she is one of the lucky ones. So much more fortunate than many of her friends. For Tom is returning uninjured — whole still, both in body and in mind.

Lately it has seemed to Ellen that everywhere she turned people were talking or writing about the "soldier to civilian" problem. Radio plays, magazine articles, newspaper stories, lecturers of all sorts, all have emphasized the changes that must be expected in the returning servicemen. She has heard it said that soldiers would seem strangers to their own families, that wives and mothers and friends would need a great deal of understanding and patience to help their men travel the long road back to happiness and usefulness in civilian life.

Hard as it is for Ellen to think of herself and Tom as among the people all this talk is about, she has tried to understand the reasons for the split between soldiers and civilians, for the bitterness that overseas veterans are said to feel about those who have stayed at home. She has read that it will be difficult to find the good-natured, happy boys who went away in the bitter, anger-hard men who come back—angry because they know the war has been bitter hard for them and at the same time know, or think, that for many people back home it has been a pleasant and profitable experience. Will Tom feel this bitterness?

Ellen has found little evidence of it in his letters, but there has been a lot of it in Bill's. Bill is her friend Mary's husband. He has been fighting in the South Pacific, and Mary has read her some of the things he wrote. "People back home seem like people beyond the grave," he said once, "so that sometimes I wonder if I want to come back at all." He called civilian problems like rationing and no cars and strikes for higher wages childish, and wrote, "We feel a certain resentment toward civilians, a resentment produced by the complete disregard of people in the States to the fact that there is a war on."

This seemed unfair to Ellen, and even to Mary. Certainly *they* knew there was a war on. *They* hadn't had such an easy time, or so they thought. Would Bill still feel this way when he got home? Would Tom? Would they come home half stranger, after a period of experience as foreign to the home folks as if they had spent it on another planet?

He may seem a stranger

Ellen is here facing a problem that many millions of women — wives, mothers, sweethearts, sisters — are facing or will face when their servicemen, some ten million of them, come home. Ellen is better off than most of them; she is aware that Tom may be different, and her recognition of this possibility will prove a good beginning if she is called upon to meet it when Tom returns.

Many women who have not done the reading, listening, and thinking that Ellen has will face the problem without recognizing it, without knowing its causes or understanding them. They have been dreaming of a life restored to "normal," of a return to the old happy companionship and mutual confidence. If they find their husbands or sons moody

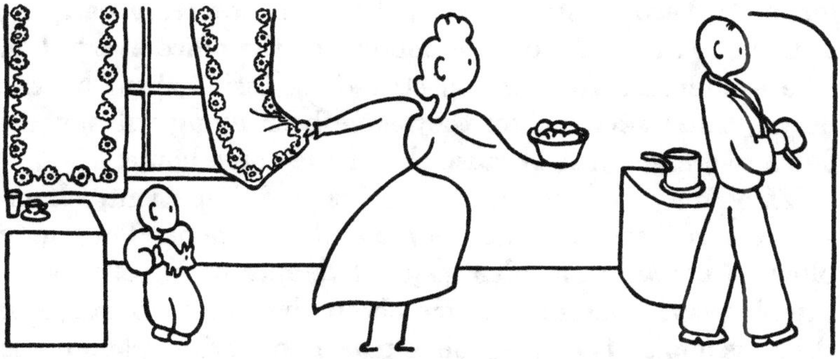

Home will be home again after a while

and restless, unconcerned about the new curtains or the old favorite pudding or even about the children, inclined to go off for walks alone or to spend their evenings with the men at the corner drugstore, they will be disappointed, bewildered, even bitter.

Understanding what is the matter will go far toward removing their heartache, understanding that for many men it will be almost as hard to come back as it was to go away. When they left they felt like the young man who wrote to his wife: "I will never forget that all-gone feeling I had when I took the oath and realized that the next few years would be dead years in my life. That day when I shucked off my nice new tweeds and came out in that wrinkled and smelly khaki uniform with clothing stickers all over the thing! Never have I felt so much like a helpless steer in a slaughter pen."

But that was three or four years ago. In the meantime, in order to endure the life and do the job demanded of them, they have either thought as little as possible about the home folks and home scenes they love so well or they have dreamed them into some ideal they never were. In either case they are likely to discover that "they have got out of the habit of living like you and me."

Some of them, it is true, will be able to settle back into old routines easily and quickly, but most of them will need longer to become steady, settled men contentedly carrying a lunch box to and from the factory or the office every day. The excitement and tension stirred up inside them by the hectic, helter-skelter lives they have been living will not die down overnight just because they have come home.

They may be nervous, explosive and impatient, chain-smokers, seekers after stimulants and diversions. They may blow off energy in sudden gusts of temper or in rough-and-tumble play. They may worry about their blood pressure or their insomnia. They may be unreasonably critical about the things you have been doing.

None of this means that they have become misfits. It simply means that they need time to get back into the swing of things. They can no more slip effortlessly back into the old life than they can blot out the memories of a thousand things the stay-at-homes have not shared with them. These memories must fade, the restlessness gradually subside.

The difficulties of readjustment will vary with the individual, according to his mental make-up and the distance he has traveled from civilian life. The greater the changes his form of service and its duration have required of him, the longer and more difficult will be the road of his return.

Consider three typical cases: John was living the relatively quiet, peaceful life of a high school teacher, seldom facing anything more frightening or violent than an unruly boy in the classroom, but the war took him to the western front in Europe. There he has lived in a foxhole for days on end, buried his dead buddy three times only to have him blown out of the earth twice in front of his eyes, has seen corpses strewn about him thick as cut grass. Dick was a garage mechanic and has spent the time behind the front lines, but in a strange land among strange people with strange customs, within sound if not sight of bursting shells and buzzing bombs. Harry was also a teacher, in a college, and he has fought the war, as he disgustedly says, "on the seat of his pants in a swivel chair" in Washington, relatively safe and comfortable.

The contribution of no one of these three is greater than that of the others; each has done his best in the task he was given. Yet no one could doubt that John has traveled farther from civilian life than Dick and Dick farther than Harry. They may return home on the same day, but it would be strange indeed if Harry did not lay aside his army experience more quickly than Dick and Dick more readily than John. But even Harry may encounter some difficulties in the process. For he too has had to submit to army discipline.

Somersaulting is not easy

The American pattern of life and education is aimed at developing individuals with strong characters, willing and wanting to think for themselves, to question and argue. Americans are proud of an "I'm from Missouri" attitude. But the first thing a soldier has to learn is to do what he is told, however unreasonable, silly, unjust, or dangerous it may seem to him. He must carry out whatever orders come from the top down, immediately and without questioning why. If he is a private he dare not go even so far as the young lieutenant whose commanding officer ordered him to grow the mustache traditionally required of British army officers.

"And mind you, none of those Charlie Chaplin affairs," said the commanding officer. "See that it's a proper mustache."

"Yes sir," the lieutenant saluted snappily. "Any particular color, sir?"

Released from the service after several years of this regimented life, this taking of orders from superiors, this following a prescribed routine in even the simplest of daily activities, the veteran will have to pick up his individual life and the responsibility for his own decisions again. Some will welcome the release and will react so violently against regimentation that they will resent the slightest advice or suggestion as to what they should do. They will seem to have a chip on their shoulder. But to knock it off will not help them, for their behavior is simply an expression of an inner need to square things with themselves for having been bossed around so long. They need a period of being undisputed captains of their own souls. If their decisions during this period are unwise and they seem to need advice, it will have to be given very tactfully indeed.

Others, those for whom decisions come hard and responsibility is a burden, will find this sudden release from regimentation difficult. In the army they have acted in concert with hundreds of other men, and something other than their own initiative has prodded them to the necessary effort. Now, out of uniform, such a man may find it difficult to get up in the morning with nothing more than an alarm clock to remind him. Every independent action, from adding up his income tax to choosing his career, may seem endless and painful. He may yearn for someone to tell him what to do, someone in authority, and he may be inclined to lean on his family or friends as he has on his sergeants, lieutenants, and captains. Such a man will have to be encouraged to stand on his own two feet once more.

A similar reaction may be the result, not of too much regimentation, but of too sudden and fearful responsibility. War may have brought the young soldier's abilities to the fore so that he was given responsibilities far beyond his years or his prewar maturity. If these have involved decisions affecting the lives of others, they may have weighed heavily upon the mind and spirit of the sensitive man.

Imagine yourself in the position of one very young sergeant. In an action in Normandy he was placed in charge of twelve men assigned to hold in the face of enemy fire a plot of ground just ten feet square. Those men and that bit of ground were his responsibility; the decisions were all his to make. He held the position but when the action was over, only three of his twelve men remained alive. Could you wonder if that young man for a time were to shrink from any decisions affecting the welfare of other persons?

An even sharper reversal demanded of a man in his adjustment to military service is in his attitude toward human life. Americans are taught and forced by law to obey the fifth commandment: Thou shalt not kill. The average boy may want to lick the daylights out of the neighborhood bully and may do so if he gets a chance, but he does not think of killing as a way of settling quarrels. Nor does anyone he knows. It is possible for most people to live a lifetime through without ever seeing anyone dead by violence.

Then suddenly the country is face to face with a dangerous international bully and the boy, trained so carefully never to kill, spends his days learning how to do that very thing in the most deadly and effective way possible. Killing has become his business, and it is the killing of men against whom he has no personal grievance, no personal anger, to help him out. Human beings, most of them, do not turn such a moral somersault without effects on their minds that it will take time to erase.

All of us, in these days of total war, have had, unconsciously at least, to change our attitude toward killing. But for those of us at home the killing has been a remote thing, not demanded of us directly. Among Americans it is the men in action at the front who, if they were to remain mentally and emotionally healthy, have had to harden themselves to accept violence and death as their daily companions.

Time for readjustment

For men in combat, life has been stripped to its raw essentials—food, sleep, and a desperate, ruthless fight for life itself. They may well need time to realize anew the importance of the pleasant little acts of grace and ceremony with which we dress these fundamentals in peacetime civilian life. Unable to count on any future, they have learned to live more intensely in the present, to snatch at any moment of delight or pleasure that offered, without heed for the consequences they might not be present to meet. For them "Eat, drink, and be merry, for tomorrow we die" has been something more real than a familiar quotation. They may have to learn all over again to take thought for the morrow, to consider consequences, to sacrifice a measure of the present for the future.

For these men in service the tempo of life has been immeasurably stepped up. For them more excitement and emotion, more action, more fear, sorrow, anger, and hate are crowded into a few days or weeks than the average civilian experiences in a lifetime. Under such compression of experience the careless, carefree boy will grow quickly into a man.

The soldier will be like a diver working in the depths of the ocean under pressure of the tremendous weight of water above him. The diver must emerge slowly to the surface when his work is done, so as to give his body time to adjust to the lessening pressure. The man returning from combat depressed and irritable, inclined to worry, to be impatient and fretful, also needs a period of decompression. He needs time for the sedative routines of civilian life to take effect and to relax the tension.

He needs these quieter pleasures, this slower life, even though he may rebel against it. Consider the boy from a simple, unpretentious home in a village or on a farm who has never been farther afield than his own state capital. In his quiet, peaceful life the greatest excitement was the weekly dance on Saturday night. Then he joins the army or the navy or the marines and sees the world. He fights and plays in far countries that were only names on a map or maybe not even that. Will it be surprising if he returns from three or four years of adventure and action to find things at home dull and monotonous, to find the dance that pleased him before the war now trivial and boring?

Imagine a pilot or a bombardier who has spent his working hours for several years in the unmarked distances of the sky. He returns home to work in a crowded city where the

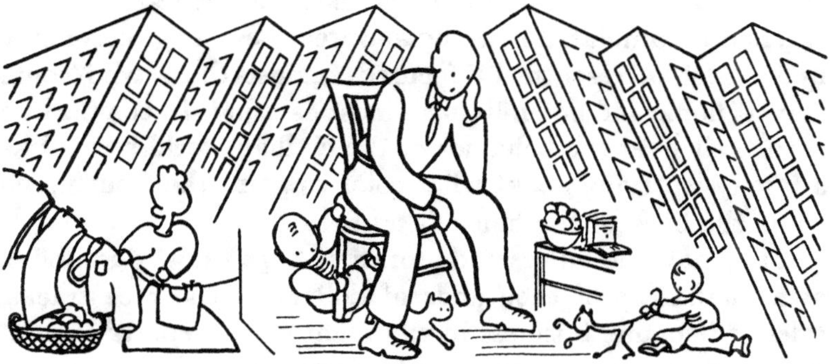

Home he's come, out of the wide blue yonder!

sky is only a narrow lane of blue between skyscraper roofs, to live in a two- or three-room apartment with his wife, the baby, and the cat. Will it be strange if he is restless, even a little wild at times with his longing for the space and freedom he knew in the air? The plea in Cole Porter's song, "Don't fence me in!" will be more than an echo in his life.

There will be all sorts of individual adjustments to be made. The man who fought the war behind the lines may feel resentful and envious if he is not honored along with the heroes of Guadalcanal by the home-town folks. Or he may feel guilty and undeserving if he is included, wondering whether he should remind them that he sat it out in Washington or London. The boy whose exploits made him a public hero for a few months will not easily accept the obscurity of an undistinguished civilian life when the world moves on to other interests.

For many soldiers the necessary adjustment will be retarded and complicated by an accumulated bitterness toward civilians. The majority of servicemen have fought the war because it had to be fought; it was a job that had to be done. This does not mean that they did not resent deeply the need for doing it, the need for interrupting their personal peacetime lives and plans. Only because they must, they have endured the mud and cold of the foxhole in Europe, the heat and insects of the jungle, the terror and tension of battle, the grief for a friend in a bomber that did not return.

Their accumulated loathing and weariness may reasonably find outlet in resentment focused against those who could stay at home and go on living almost as usual. In comparison with their lives the behavior of the civilian world seems like a family worrying about what color to paint the front porch while the back of the house is on fire.

They have heard or read stories of huge crowds gambling away hundreds of thousands of dollars at the race tracks, tales of booming business in gay night clubs, reports of jam-packed department stores and tremendous stocks sold out at fabulous prices at Christmastime. And all this was happening on the very same day that they were staking their lives to gain and hold a beachhead in Normandy. Or the same day that they were leaving half their number dead on the sands of Tarawa. Or the very same Christmastime when they were trying desperately to beat back a crucial German counter-offensive in Belgium.

Under such glaring disparities can the servicemen be expected to remember that they have only a part of the picture, that these facts are not the whole of the civilian story?

Need for a two-way understanding

If Tom comes home with any of these problems or another like them in origin — and he will almost certainly do so — Ellen, his parents, and his friends should understand that there is nothing abnormal or mysterious in his attitude. The transition from soldier to civilian is a variation of the normal, ordinary adjustments human beings have to make in the course of life. The depressed and irritable serviceman is going through the process often seen in persons who have passed through a great grief or personal crisis. The war hero who feels let down when the public begins to forget him is like the football hero who must get used to being inconspicuous after he has left the gridiron. The veteran with a chip on his shoulder is kin to the man bossed by his wife at home who seeks to square things with himself by bossing everyone in sight at the office or the factory.

The problem, then, is a natural one and is to be expected under the circumstances. What is needed to meet it most effectively is a two-way understanding: an understanding of the man's plight and needs on the part of the family and friends, and on the part of the man himself an understanding of his own feelings and of the civilian world to which he has returned.

The women must realize that their men are not just being cussed, mean, contrary, difficult; that there is a very good reason for their behavior, even though they themselves do not understand what is wrong. They may only know that coming home does not give them the perfect happiness they dreamed it would, that something is missing which leaves them restless and dissatisfied.

If the man is restless and bitter, snapping at the wife he idealized when he was overseas, if he longs for companionship and then shies away from it, the wife must realize that his behavior is a silent cry for help. It means that he, like everyone, is groping for a path in the face of difficulties. He is trying to find his balance again, to reconcile his ambitions, desires, and needs with the necessity for socially effective living. He is lonely and confused. He feels out of place in the life he has returned to, longing and needing to get in step with it, but not knowing how.

Some do's and don'ts

Welcome him home and enjoy his company. Evidence that his presence is enjoyed is more reassuring than pity.

Listen well. Listen to as much or as little as he wishes to tell. So much was said after the last war about the "silent soldier," the boy who refused to talk about the battles he had seen, that many families or friends may be unnaturally self-conscious on the subject. They may recount tediously all the accumulated neighborhood gossip in an attempt to avoid the subject they imagine the soldier will not want to talk about—until *their* soldier, who *wants* to talk, feels that they are not interested in what has happened to him. He may be the kind that feels that to go through a major battle and come out alive is something to talk about.

How men can joke in the midst of misery and danger, can sit on a hilltop while artillery shells are flying overhead and calmly describe the whistling projectiles as "incoming" or "outgoing," *is* something to talk about. But no two men react alike. While some gain a certain relief by "spilling" it, instinctively knowing that it is better to uncork painful memories than to try to bury them, others need the comfort of silence and will want just to sit in the sun smoking and thinking.

Make sure that you give your serviceman a chance to tell about his army life, but do not pry. If he wants to talk he will, and if he doesn't, all right. Don't urge him.

Be natural and casual. Think of him as an individual, not a veteran; as a man, not a case. Do not let too much over-dramatization, too many headlines screaming "All Veterans Seen as Problems," rob you of your common sense. Do not see a problem where none exists; do not begin looking for problems in every returned soldier you see or hear about.

Do not set him apart because of his military experiences. Emphasis upon his differences, the greatness of his sacrifices, the horror or heroism of his experiences is highly undesirable. Pity will do him more harm than neglect. Try to understand the struggle he is going through, but do not coddle him in his difficulties. For his own happiness and mental health, he must get back to normal civilian attitudes and activities as quickly as the necessary adjustment permits.

Do not fuss over him too much. Don't try to cater to his slightest whim. The family might learn a lesson here from the fact that military hospital authorities and army doctors prefer not to have parents visit the wounded boys because the patients are so often restless afterward and their recovery is retarded.

Fathers are said to be worse in this regard than mothers. They seem more upset; in their love and anxiety they want to do so much for their boy that they get in their own way and his. The father who fusses about whether the cigarettes are close enough for the boy to reach is trying to ease his own feelings more than to ensure the patient's comfort. If the boy wants the cigarettes he will reach for them or ask to have them handed to him.

Be patient with him. Getting accustomed to civilian schedules may not be easy, and he may have undergone emotional and personality changes. Encourage him to take up hobbies and be normally active in social life—with old friends and new. But do not make a point of it.

Especially irritating to anyone suffering from nerves, anyone feeling out of tune, is the eternal nagging "why?" Why don't you sit down? Why don't you talk? Why don't you eat your cake; isn't it made the way you like it? A person who is already conscious that he is not doing what is expected of him, he scarcely knows why not, may be driven by such a barrage of questions to the point of wanting to shout in answer, "Why don't you go to hell?"

The difficulty in many cases is that the relatives and friends are considering themselves, not the returned serviceman. Their lives since he went away have been days of waiting, and they want to celebrate his return. So they arrange a family party or they invite the neighbors in to rejoice with them over the traveler's safe return. Naturally they are disappointed if he is not spontaneously and wholeheartedly happy about it. It's all in his honor; it's all for him. Why doesn't he enjoy it? Isn't he glad to be home again? What's the matter with him?

Nothing. He should and will resume his participation in social life, but he may not be ready to do it the evening he returns, or the next day, the next week, or the next month. Give him time to get used to home and let him feel a steadfast understanding upon which he can depend even when he seems most illogical and resentful.

Remember always that his actions are not personal slights, however much they may seem so. The mother who has spent all day in a hot kitchen in order to serve her boy his favorite dinner on his first night at home, should not take it personally if he eats little or nothing. She should not be sure that her culinary skill has failed her just when she wanted it most, that her boy doesn't like her cooking any more. Her boy is probably only too aware that he is disappointing his mother, and her disappointment repeatedly expressed will only make him feel worse.

If in the midst of a family party he goes off for a walk alone, the family may naturally be disappointed because after so long an absence they want him with them. But there is nothing personal in his going off; it does not mean that he doesn't love his family any more, that he doesn't enjoy being with them. Let him walk off his restlessness in the wind and rain, and when he returns welcome him back naturally and casually.

He must do his part

The process of adjustment will proceed faster and smoother if the veteran also understands what his difficulty is and what is required of him: to pick up again as soon as he can the simpler, less exciting, seemingly less important routines of civilian life. He should realize that the upheaval he has passed through is something extraordinary in human affairs and that its continuance is neither possible nor desirable. Few individuals can or should live their lives through on the plane of intensity on which he has lived for the past years. For his own health and happiness, as well as those of his family, his job now is to relax, to let the tension go from his mind, his nerves, his muscles.

This is not an easy task, but it may help him to remember that "the longest journey begins with a single step." The singer Chaliapin used to put this old proverb to very practical use. He needed the exercise of walking home from downtown New York, but the sixty blocks to his hotel seemed too wearying in prospect. So he started out to walk, never the whole sixty blocks, but just five blocks to a shooting gallery he knew on Sixth Street. After watching a few people miss the bull's-eye there, he started on the eleven blocks to Carnegie Hall, where it fascinated him to study the faces of the people buying tickets for the evening's performance. Tiring of that pastime, he set out on the eight blocks to the Central Park Zoo, to get a chuckle out of a gorilla that looked very like a certain tenor he knew and didn't like much.

In this way he progressed in easy, pleasant stages, and his sixty blocks were covered almost before he knew it. He once summarized his walk in this way: "It is a lesson in the art of living. Never worry about the distance between you and your goal. Always concentrate on what is within five short blocks from you. Don't let the faraway future bother you. Always think of the joys, no matter how small, awaiting you in the next twenty-four hours."

For the veteran, the "five short blocks" may be just an hour's visit from Mrs. Grundy who lives next door, or an evening with Aunt Sally who treats him like the little boy he was in the days on which her memory dwells. Or it may be a dance with his old gang who now seem silly and immature. He should try to remember how he used to take these occasions in his stride, without strain or distress, even with amusement and active pleasure. He will do so again once he gets the feel of things, once the habits and ways of reacting he formed in the army give way to habits and reactions more suitable for civilian life.

Let him try to remember that the actions and remarks of the people around him are seldom meant as personal slights or insinuations. If he fought in Italy and his barber insists that the action in France was more important and more heroic, instead of feeling himself unappreciated and misun-

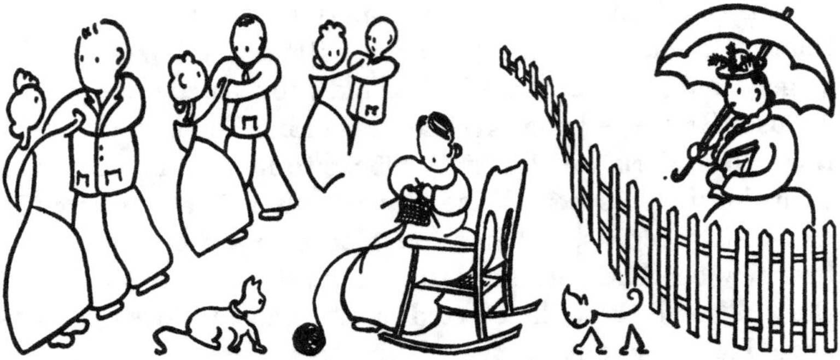

He will take them in his stride again

derstood he should understand that the barber is only trying to console himself by enhancing the contribution of his son, who died in France. Perhaps the barber should take a broader view, but most of us see the world between the blinders of our own experience.

After all, the veteran may be looking at the world with blinders of his own. If he finds his wife's chatter about a chipped fingernail a bit galling because he recalls women he saw crawling across a battlefield under fire to drag back wounded men, he must realize that his wife is not on a battlefield with wounded men needing care. If she were, she might well rise to the same heights of courage as the women he remembers.

If he is sour and cynical about the civilians who spent the war in continued comfort and safety, he must try to understand that most of them did the best they could in the things demanded of them. Against all the talk of strikes, high wages, absenteeism, and the like, stands the indisputable fact of a miracle of production, which made possible in no small measure his victory and his safe return.

He might recover a truer perspective if he could realize that the dull monotony of waiting, the slow drain of worry, unrelieved by any opportunity for direct, tangible action toward ending the struggle, requires a fortitude and stamina of its own, less dramatic and less obvious than those the soldier needs but nevertheless telling in its toll of nervous strength.

But if the veteran is too sunk in bitter regrets and self-pity to see these truths, it will help neither you nor him to argue the matter. Simply point out that however hard and unjust his lot was in comparison with those who stayed at home, it does him no good to go on moaning about it. Feeling sorry for himself won't put the spilled milk back into the pitcher. His regrets and recriminations, whether justified or not, are just wasting his time. He has returned to the civilian world and he must live in it, so the sooner he accepts its ways and standards again, the better off he will be.

And it will save him heartache in the end if he realizes in the beginning that the public will not long remember, at least not to the point of special consideration, the men who fought and bled for them. They will become too involved with the problems of today and tomorrow to give more than an occasional passing thought to yesterday's war and its heroes and its victims.

Right or wrong, this is the world's way. It does not linger long in the past; it moves on. And the veteran, to be a happy and effective person, must forget that he is a veteran and move on with it. He has done his job in the war, done it well; his job now is to do as well in the peacetime world.

He must recognize the source of much of his resentment: the soldier is not angry at the civilian because he is a civilian, but because the civilian has a way of life that the soldier wants. In the same way many civilians resent the soldier because he was in the fight when they feel they were not.

But it never does any good to resent the good fortune of others. If a person gets hit by an automobile and is injured, it will not help him any to be angry at the people who did not get hit. The soldier must recognize that either because of his own ideals or because he just happened to be in a certain age group he got "hit" by the army. He had to fight society's war, a war that he feels was not of his making—which is good cause for resentment. But the only way such resentment can benefit him or anyone else is to energize it toward an aggressive peace. Let him take his place as a member of society and direct his energies toward preventing wars in the future.

All this and marriage too

The restlessness and impatience produced by the transition to civilian life will also surround and complicate the more personal adjustments that everyday living requires of the individual. For instance, consider Ellen and Tom, whose story we have told. Ellen is aware of the general problem we have been discussing, but she is not aware that she and Tom have still to face their individual problem—the normal adjustments of married life. She and Tom have still to work out the routines and details of their life together, which will be the real test of their compatibility and their maturity.

Marriage at any time requires the formation of new habits in relation to another's ways and rights. Each partner in a successful marriage must be prepared to give as well as take. Each must be willing to forgo a measure of the personal freedom he has enjoyed in compensation for the companionship and love he will gain.

Under ordinary circumstances, adjustment is facilitated by the fact that the pattern of American society as well as the needs and desires of most individuals makes marriage the normal and ideal state. In any desirable change we are likely not to mind little annoyances. We will cheerfully knock our shins against the crowded furniture of a stuffy hotel room because there is such a nice view from the window of that room. So in looking through the window of society, where marriage presents such a fine view, minor annoyances are accepted without the individual's realizing what is happening.

So in the average marriage, because it is a new situation and a socially desirable one, new habits are formed and substituted for old ones gradually and painlessly. This is true especially when the people are young and eager for change.

But with Ellen and Tom these new marriage habits are not yet formed. Although they knew each other fairly well before their marriage, they will find that there is a good deal they have not known. Ellen may know that Tom likes to drive fast in a car, but she does not know how he will act when he has no car to drive. She knows that he likes to tinker with automobiles, but she has yet to learn how he will react to news that the faucet is broken, or the lamp, or the window. She knows that he is careful about his appearance and always looks well dressed, but she does not know in what condition he leaves his bedroom in the process. These things she must learn and adjust to.

Also, Ellen has much to learn about herself. Although she has been married three years and has a two-year-old child, she has not yet experienced the pleasures and pains of home-making. Will she learn to cook well and do it three times a day? Will she wince or even protest aloud every time Tom misses the ash tray? If he's the sort that strews his belongings from front to back of the apartment, with stopovers at every possible point between, how will she take it?

If she finds herself inclined to be the kind of wife who puts the state of the house above the comfort of the family, she will do well to make a change in herself. She must learn to get satisfaction from creating order anew each day out of the chaos Tom and Tommy leave behind. And if this does not satisfy her passion for neatness, she can work it off in side-lines—like the wife who kept lovebirds and took out her reforming instincts on them instead of her husband. Their dexterity in slinging birdseed over the deep-piled carpet proved a good match for this passion in her.

Or perhaps Ellen will find that she is not cut out to be a housekeeper. She may greatly prefer to go on working in an office. Nonetheless she has taken on the job of making a home for Tom and Tommy, and her personal problem must be solved with full consideration for this obligation to the comfort and happiness of these two others.

The children

Tommy himself may prove a complicating factor that Ellen has not counted on. She may proudly plant a two-year-old child on Tom's knee, fully expecting him to be overjoyed by this product of his paternity, to find instead that he behaves as if his collar were choking him.

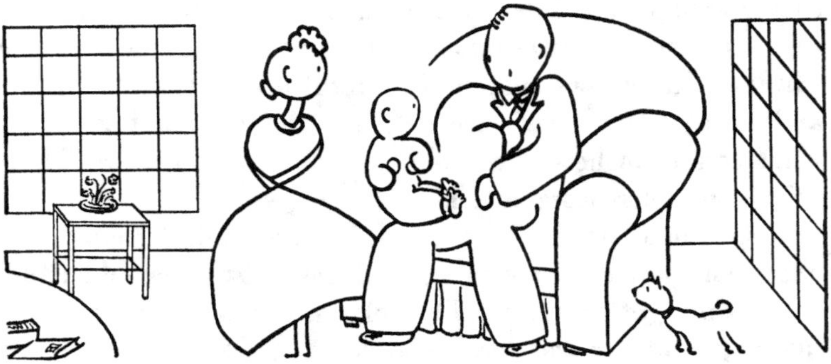

Little stranger

Yes, of course Tom knows all about Tommy. He has been proud and pleased to show his buddies the pictures Ellen sent him and to read them reports of the youngster's progress. "Gee, imagine me having a kid back home," he often said to himself and to them. But he has also been dreaming of all the things he and Ellen would do together when he got home. Especially when his pals, first one and then another, were sent out of England — to Africa, to Italy, to Paris — and he had to stay behind, he consoled himself with thoughts of all the places he and Ellen would go when he got home.

What Tom probably has not done is to fit his two dreams together and reconcile the conflict between them. He hasn't counted on Ellen's eternal "I can't, because of Tommy." This continual interference with his plans will take some getting used to, and there will be arguments and misunderstandings in the process. Under the most favorable circumstances a first child raises new problems in marriage, and if the child is two years old when the father first makes its acquaintance, these problems are likely to be aggravated.

If she must face this situation, Ellen should realize that there is nothing monstrous or unnatural in Tom's attitude. Being Tommy's father will not automatically and immediately make him love the child and accept willingly its demands upon him. The love of parents for children and of children for parents is based much more on shared associations and experiences and mutual interdependence than on the blood relationship.

Just as a successful, happy marriage is built up only through months and years of shared living and responsibility, so a feeling of belongingness comes only through the experience of belonging. Unless Ellen and Tom recognize the importance of this feeling and take special care to develop it in their son, Tommy will be numbered among the casualties of this war. Like other war babies born into homes not yet established, Tommy has never had the chance to develop a feeling of belonging to anybody or to any place. Shuttled between grandmothers by day, seeing his mother only at night, Tommy has felt the winds of authority blow from many different directions.

Unless Ellen and Tom take special steps to make a place for Tommy in both their lives, he will continue to feel an outsider. Particularly when a second child is born, they must take special care to make Tommy feel a part of the family. If not, his experience will be like that of the illegitimate child whose mother later marries and takes him into her new home. Other children are born who belong naturally in the family, but the first child never quite belongs; he lives forever a shadow on the outskirts of the home.

Tommy may be a war casualty in another sense too. Tom, like so many other servicemen in the transition from army to civilian life, may for a time be a member of the No-back-talk-from-a-kid-of-mine school. He may take the attitude that Tommy should "toe the line," that he should "learn straight off to do what he's told *when* he's told." If Tom tends to feel this way, both he and Ellen should recognize what is at work; he has a hangover from army discipline. They must both work to make sure that Tommy doesn't suffer from the effects of his father's experience with a top sergeant.

War brides

Such domestic problems may be greatly increased if the waiting wife is even more of a "war bride" than Ellen—that is, if the total acquaintance of the couple has been limited to three weeks or perhaps even three days. With the glamour of the uniform gone, they may find each other less attractive as life partners than they thought when they were under the influence of the unnatural excitement of war. On such short acquaintance their feelings may have been a passing fancy.

After a long separation the one can hardly remember what the other looks like; interest has waned and the marriage seems like a dream. The husband cannot forget because his pay checks have become smaller—the family allotment and insurance each month is a firm reminder of his postwar responsibilities. The partners in such a marriage may well seem strangers to each other. And unless their reunion can take on many of the characteristics of a genuine courtship, much disappointment and disharmony will occur.

A fair proportion of such war marriages may prove unworkable and will have to be numbered among the casualties of the war. But this is by no means true of all of them, or even of the majority, if the persons involved are mature, intelligent persons, with a realistic view of marriage instead of some vague romantic notions about it—if they know that marriage at best requires a goodly amount of willing effort on both sides to make it work.

The danger is that with their undue haste to serve as a good alibi, these war brides and grooms will not try hard enough for success, that they will give up before they are really licked. They may mistake the normal problems of marriage for evidences of incompatibility just because they know so well how slight was the acquaintance on which they married. The real war bride faces a task that will challenge her intelligence, adaptability, and tact to the full, but if she wants to make her marriage a success, she probably can. Both she and her husband must recognize that the first weeks of his return are *not* the normal situation out of which they should judge each other. They must both have time to evaluate their relationship, to develop mutual understanding, tolerance, cooperation, and compromise. Otherwise they will begin asking themselves, "How could I have married anyone who behaves like this?"

Wives of longer standing

Somewhat different is the case of the couple whose marriage was of several years' standing before the war interrupted it. For them, the adjustments had been made, the habits formed. And the chances are that once the husband has accepted his return to civilian life, these two will find themselves back on the old footing. The war will have changed few of their leopard's spots; it will have turned few household devils into angels or vice versa.

But for a time even they may find themselves strangers in some ways and will need to get acquainted all over again. If so, the adjustments will not be so easy as when they were newly married. Each may have acquired characteristics with which the other does not know how to deal. The soldier, walking out his dreary sentry duty, humming softly "Home on the Range," dreams of his wife as young, pretty, gay, lighthearted. It may be a shock when he comes home to find her sober, mature, not very playful, looking older than she is. And he on his part may have turned from a handsome, gay, energetic person to a haggard, preoccupied, now grim and tired husband.

Here again the problem of personal freedom may enter the picture. The husband has had to break his home habits and form new ones in keeping with army life. He has regained the freedom of his bachelor days, or an even greater freedom perhaps, for as a bachelor he may still have been under his mother's thumb. But in the army, once his day was finished and he was off duty, no one asked him where he was going or when he would be back. So he spent his Saturday nights or free weekends in his own way, and after several years of this he may just have got out of the habit of the usual courtesy of saying where he is going when he leaves the house.

The wife too may have got used to being more independent, especially the wife who has been working in an office or a factory. However fond she is of her husband, she may find herself reluctant to give up the pleasure of organizing her life as it suits her without having to plan almost every hour of it around him.

These are natural reactions and should be recognized as such. They are nothing to feel guilty about, nothing about which to reproach either one's self or the other. Give each other time and in most cases the old habits of mutual dependence and confidence will be re-established.

If for some time to come, the husband seems to prefer the company of other ex-soldiers to that of his wife or his family, the wife should not allow herself to be jealous. It does not mean that their marriage is going on the rocks.

For months or years now the husband has been a member of a closely knit group of men. Working and playing with them, sharing responsibility, danger, and death with them, he has come, quite unconsciously no doubt, to draw strength and support from their mutual and collective loyalties. More than that, his very life has been in their hands, and their lives in his; the safety of each has depended on the close teamwork of all. Psychologists tell us that to lose the sustaining force of such a group relationship will create an emotional problem for almost any individual.

So the veteran's wife must be prepared to have her husband feel more at ease for a time with men who have shared his or similar experiences. It is a natural reaction. The men speak his language at the moment, and they understand what he is going through because they are having the same difficulties. In time he will again have civilian language and civilian experiences to relate, and will gradually find the companionship of his family more and more satisfying.

For some time, and perhaps indefinitely, he may want to keep in touch with his veteran friends and join one or more of the service organizations. He will become interested in their activities and will very likely soon ask his wife to join the auxiliary of whatever organization he has chosen. Thus will be established an important social outlet for them both. Each year they will look forward to the district, state, or national meetings. The people they meet will become mutual friends, for they will all have interests *and* experiences in common.

No apron strings

What of the men who return unmarried? Since eighteen to twenty is the commonest age of soldiers in this war, the majority of them will probably be returning to mothers instead of to wives.

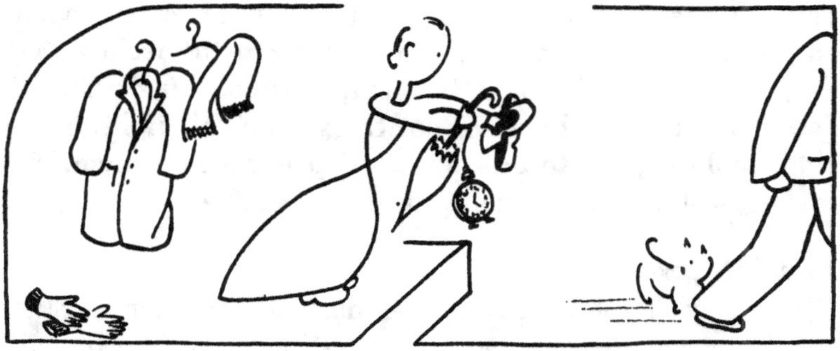

Cut those apron strings

Here the most common problem will be for the mother to realize that her little boy has grown up. In her mind he will have remained as he was when he went away, the immature boy who was guided by family opinions, family decisions, and family instructions. But the experiences he has undergone have probably matured him into a man, wanting to live his own life and in most cases capable of doing so. He may not submit so patiently as he did to being told when to wear his rubbers or his muffler, what time to get in at night, what companions he should have, and so on.

Parents who try to take up with their son where they left off, who infringe upon his hard-won and deserved independence of action, are just heading for trouble. Instead they must recognize his right to live his own life in his own way, however far that seems from their way.

In some cases this recognition may be complicated by the fact that the boy's wisdom really does not match his wish for independence. In the army he has been independent of his parents financially as well as mentally and morally, but this independence has not been of a kind to develop good habits in the management of money. What pay he received he was free to spend as frivolously or recklessly as he liked; his essential needs in food, clothes, and medical care were automatically provided. It may not be easy for him to learn all at once how to provide these necessities for himself, and until he does he may become temporarily dependent again on his family. This in turn may give them the feeling that they again have the right to dictate his course. Perhaps it does, but they will be wiser not to exercise this right. Their aim should be, not to broaden his dependence on them, but to narrow it as much and as quickly as possible.

The job problem

Along with these general and domestic problems, Ellen and Tom will have to face the question of their economic future. What is Tom to do to support the family he has now acquired? Of the possibilities open to him, which shall he choose?

The law says that he may have his old job back if he wants it, and since Tom went into service early, there will probably be little question about his title to the job. But suppose the firm he worked for, under the pressure of wartime production needs, has completely reorganized its setup, or under the limitations of rationing and shortages has gone out of business entirely, so that Tom's job no longer exists.

What is Tom to do then? Or if the job still exists and Tom chooses to take it back, what are Ned and Alf to do, the two men who succeeded Tom in turn before they were drafted?

In these cases the re-employment committee of the selective service board or the veterans' employment representative of the United States Employment Service (USES) will do their best to find the men jobs equivalent to the one they left. The law on this matter cannot be applied according to its exact letter; practical circumstances will not permit. It must be interpreted in its spirit, with common sense and perhaps compromise on all sides.

Many returned servicemen, however, will not want their old jobs back; they will want better ones. Take the case of the eighteen-year-old who was a copy boy in a newspaper office when he was drafted. In the army he has risen to the rank of sergeant. He almost certainly will not be content to return to the status of copy boy. Or consider the youthful account clerk who has been charged with increasing responsibility for organizing vast and intricate networks of supply in the navy. The subordinate position and the unchallenging routines of his old job may be intolerable to him.

Complications will arise when the men who want jobs in keeping with their greater maturity are not technically qualified for more advanced positions. Having become a flight commander does not make a man a better bookkeeper, but it will almost certainly have made him want a better job. And when his former employer cannot give him the better job because he is not qualified to hold it, he will, naturally and humanly, take out his frustration in resentment against men who stayed at home and with increasing experience and training were promoted to the higher positions and salaries he wants too. He will feel that he has lost out, unfairly, by his years of service to his country.

To be emotionally mature but to lack the training and experience for a more responsible economic role is bound to create strain and frustration. But railing and ranting about what might have been or what ought to have been will not change matters. Proclaiming loudly to all who pass that one has been abused may relieve a bit of internal pressure, but it will do no further good.

Less upsetting perhaps but equally pressing are the job problems of the men who went into the army straight from high school without holding a job to go back to, and also of the men whom army tests have shown to have abilities and aptitudes unsuited to the work they were doing.

For all these men two practical alternatives are possible. They may take advantage of the schooling benefits offered by the GI Bill of Rights, or they may make use of the special job-placement service offered them by the USES.

His for the asking

If they wish to acquire the training they need for a better or a different job, the government will pay for it and will also pay them enough to live on while they are studying. If the discharged serviceman does not already know the details of this generous offer or how they apply in his case, he has only to write or call at the nearest office of the Veterans Administration or one of the various organizations given on pages 35 to 37.

There are cases on record that show what this education benefit can mean to the veteran. One man was a taxicab driver before he enlisted. His army adviser found that he rated very high in literary and scientific aptitudes, so when he received his medical discharge he enrolled at his state university to train himself for high school teaching. Another man did not want to return to his job of theater doorman and so is learning to be an upholsterer.

One young farmer in the army tests displayed a manipulative ability 99 per cent higher than that of the general public. He is now apprenticed to a big metropolitan optical company, where he is learning to use his clever fingers in the fine skills of an optician finisher. And a former magazine salesman is gratifying through this training benefit a lifelong ambition to learn the intricacies of bookkeeping.

This opportunity for education in some specific profession or skilled craftsmanship is so obviously worth while that no veteran entitled to it should pass it by without careful consideration. Above all, he ought not to throw it away because at the moment he feels he cannot possibly stand the discipline of study, the concentrated practice needed to learn a new skill, or the imagined humiliation of going back to school at his age, perhaps in classes of men and women younger and much less mature than himself. Teachers and school administrators are aware of these special problems, and in most cases reasonable allowances will be made in requirements and regulations for the older, more responsible student. In any case, an education or a course of training in some technical field is well worth the cost it may entail in petty irritations or annoyances.

But in many cases individual circumstances or inclinations may make this benefit unattractive or out of the question. Then the man's aim should be to find the kind of work best suited to his abilities and most likely to make use of the training and experience he has had in the army. There probably won't be any civilian job exactly like his army job. Where, then, can he find out what kind of civilian job will use his particular skills?

At the local office of the USES. Each of these offices has special counselors and interviewers charged with the task of placing veterans in satisfactory jobs. And these staff members have on their desks copies of a 500-page book specially prepared to meet this problem by the War Manpower Commission in cooperation with the army and the navy. This book lists 23,000 civilian jobs grouped in families related to one another in the skills or knowledge they require. And each "job family" is compared to some definite army or navy job.

Here is an example of how the USES advisers will use this book as a guide in finding work for the men who come for placement: John Doe doesn't want to go back to his civilian job of shipping clerk. In the army he was trained to be an airplane armorer gunner and he wants some peacetime work similar to that. The job-family book will tell the adviser that John Doe can be a testing-machine operator, a gas-meter repairman, a vending-machine assembler, or perhaps a gunsmith. These are the civilian jobs that most nearly resemble his army job, and in one of these the USES man will try to place him.

To change or not to change

It may not be easy for the veteran to fit into the job found for him, however well it may suit his abilities. The transition restlessness that is complicating all phases of his life at the moment may plague him here too. He may feel more or less like the man whose service in the navy has taken him all over the seven seas but whose civilian job as a responsible executive keeps him in an office all day long. He is upset because he feels he just can't sit at a desk all day; he can't concentrate on his work. He feels he will simply blow up, sitting within the same four walls all the time. He is an intelligent man and he knows the work he is doing is important. If he gives it a chance, and gives himself some time to readjust, he will work into it all right. In the meantime, when the pressure gets too great, he had better take a day off and go fishing, golfing, or hiking in the open air.

Many men, if they are not careful, will fall victim to the old and common "greener pastures" complex. Something else will always seem better, more desirable, to them than what they have. They will become dissatisfied with the job they have and think there are better jobs paying more money in some other plant, some other office, or some other part of the country. They will be sure that they would be happier working somewhere else. So they will quit their job and take another, only to find that they have carried their restlessness with them and are no happier in the new position than in the old.

Unless and until these men realize that the trouble lies within themselves and so will accompany them wherever they go, they may move from one job to another all over the country, never coming to grips with any job, never giving themselves a chance to master any skill. This is what ails many of the "job hobos" of peacetime as well as war.

To decide whether one is justified in making a change or is simply yielding to this transient restlessness will require honest self-analysis and thoughtful investigation of the factors involved. And it may call for equal honesty, wisdom, even self-sacrifice, on the part of the man's family.

Take the case of the young man who went to war from an Iowa farm. He seems to be good at farming, and so far as anyone, including himself, knows, he means to be a farmer for life. While he is away his parents do what they have always dreamed of doing; they buy him a farm, so that he will have something safe and sure to come back to.

But in the meantime their son has tasted another kind of life. In the army signal corps he has shown a special aptitude for photography, has been given a great deal of training in it, and has proved highly successful in practicing it. He has found too that he likes people, enjoys meeting them and getting around among them. He does not want to go back to the loneliness of the farm; he wants now to become a newspaper photographer.

The chances are in this case that the man's choice is a wise one, but it will certainly hurt his parents. It will take him off to the city, away from them. It will wreck the dreams they have built in these lonely years of waiting for his return. Nevertheless, they ought to realize that the intensity of their disappointment comes of their having dreamed and acted according to their own wishes, not his. It is for them now to yield to his decision, and to do so in such a way that he need not feel guilty for refusing their gift and going on about his own life.

Very different is the problem of the young man who was a clerk in a hardware store in a small South Dakota town.

He has not distinguished himself in any way in the army, nor has he learned any new skills. But he has stood in the glitter of bright lights on Broadway, has felt himself a man of the world on weekend sprees in Paris, has licked his lips in envy of those of his buddies who can match "lines" with the "slick chicks" that work in city offices. And so as his homeward train carries him through the farmlands and small towns of middle America, he says to himself: How do people stand it living there? How do they get on, when nothing exciting ever happens? They can't have any fun. This man will not willingly settle down to the life he left. He too will want to go off to the city to live. Perhaps he should try the change, but the chances are that he will be neither happy nor successful if he does.

Psychological tension is always the result of conflict between desires and attainments. This man's desires have been greatly increased by his army experiences, but his ability to attain those desires may *not* have increased. If it has not, until he recognizes and accepts the fact that however much he may want the glitter of urban sophistication, he does not have it and would not be really happy in it, he is in for some bad moments of strain and frustration.

Some returned servicemen, not many we hope, will lean heavily on the idea that the world owes them a living. If things get tough, or even if they don't, these men will excuse themselves from responsibility and effort by feeling that in risking their lives in military combat they have discharged their obligations to society once and for all. It is true that society owes them an incalculable debt, but they will be farther ahead in mental health and happiness if they never seek payment in coin other than the opportunity to make for themselves the best living of which they are capable.

If despite everyone's best efforts the returned serviceman cannot find a job, the GI Bill of Rights guarantees him unemployment compensation for a maximum of fifty-two weeks. But he will do well not to rest too contentedly on this proffered cushion. His future, like everyone else's, depends on the future of the country, on the establishment of a prosperous civilian economy. Things have not changed in this respect while he was away, and it will still be necessary for him to pitch in and help make the wheels go round if he wants to live on something more satisfactory than the dole.

You are not alone

Whichever of these problems Ellen and Tom face, they will not have to solve them alone and unaided. They will, of course, have to make their own final decisions; no one can do that for them. But they can get good advice and information to help them choose wisely.

Because there will be so many Ellens and Toms when the war is over, their readjustments constitute a general social problem as well as a personal one. It is to the advantage of all of us that the returned servicemen fit back into civilian life as quickly, as painlessly, and as effectively as possible. It is for this reason, to reduce both the individual and the social cost of readjustment and reconversion, that various governmental agencies, both federal and local, have been set up to provide information and guidance to the veterans and their families.

We have already mentioned the services offered by the USES, one of the federal agencies, but there are many other organizations ready to give almost any kind of help or service that is needed.

There is, of course, the Veterans Administration, a federal government agency charged with the administration of all veterans' affairs. All questions of benefits under the GI Bill of Rights, disability pensions, vocational retraining, and the like are referred to this government bureau. But if there is no Veterans Administration office near your home you may seek advice from one of several other agencies.

There is, first of all, the American Red Cross, which now has a chapter or branch in every county in the country. The Red Cross is the agent of the American people, who support it by voluntary contributions. Its services, which include

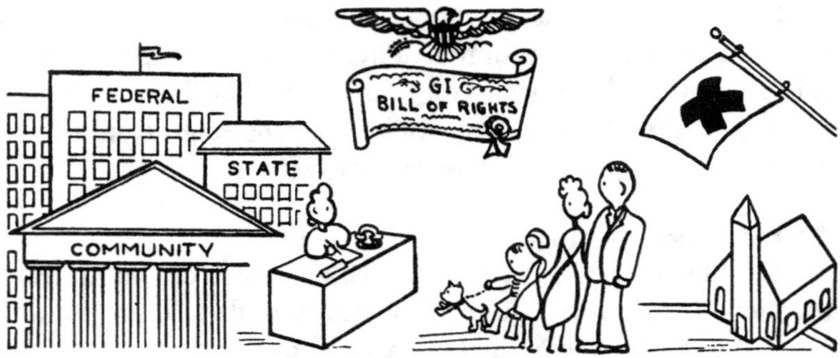

You are not alone

everything from advice on personal problems to a financial lift in an emergency, are nonpolitical, nonsectarian, and without race or sex limitations. Since the Red Cross is both a national and international organization, applicants for assistance need not be residents of any particular area or members of any particular organization.

Also ready to help the veteran and his family are the various service organizations, of which the American Legion, the Disabled American Veterans, and the Veterans of Foreign Wars are the chief ones. In practically every city, town, and hamlet in the United States you will find an active representative, called a service officer, of one or all of these organizations. In the larger cities they have staffs of both paid and volunteer workers to assist the veteran, and, like the Red Cross, they render a wide variety of services, including both guidance and financial assistance when necessary. Their services, however, are available only to their own members, or to the members of their women's auxiliary groups.

There are also various state and city agencies, such as state departments of veterans' affairs, family welfare agencies, and other such units grouped in the Council of Social Agencies and financed by community funds. In most cities and towns, too, there are branches of one or more of the organizations that comprise the USO—the YMCA, YWCA, Salvation Army, National Catholic Community Service, Jewish Welfare Board, and National Travelers Aid Association —all of which offer special services.

The YMCA, for example, offers three months free membership to all returned veterans, with the hope and purpose of providing facilities for group recreation that will help servicemen bridge the gap between army and civilian life. Servicemen who have come to feel a certain security from being an integral part of an army or navy group must develop new patterns of loyalty and security in civilian groups. It is during this transition period that such organizations as the YMCA can help if the servicemen give them the chance.

These are only a few of the agencies whose services are available to the veteran. Because there are so many of them, few persons know enough about them to select quickly and correctly the one that can help them best. Recognizing this fact, the War Manpower Commission has set up in each community a Veterans Service Committee, whose job it is to centralize and coordinate the work of all the various agencies. It is to this committee that the veteran who needs help of any kind and doesn't know where to find it should go. If he cannot locate this committee, his selective service board can direct him to it.

In the larger communities the service committees are establishing Veterans Information Centers to which the veteran or his family may go for advice, without wandering all over town seeking for the help they need. These centers are staffed with expert interviewers and counselors—mostly ex-servicemen themselves—who are acquainted with all the manifold difficulties that are likely to confront the serviceman and also with all the complicated machinery available to help him. When they learn what his problems are they will know what agency and what person in it can best help him. They will make an appointment for him so that he can go there and get in quickly without loss of time, without more of the endless waiting in line that has irked him so in the army.

Take it or leave it

It is quite possible that the veteran himself will scorn all this assistance that is available to him. He thinks he's all right. He knows what he wants to do, or at least what he ought to do. Why should he go off downtown to ask some stranger for advice? Besides, he's tired of being questioned and tested and talked to about what he should do. He's going to make up his own mind for a change.

It may be well worth the family's while to persuade him out of this attitude if possible. Point out that no one will try to make up his mind for him; the aim of the counselors provided is merely to give him information and suggestions. When his decisions at this point mean so much for his future, why not take what assistance is offered, why not see what light an outsider — with special knowledge and experience — can cast upon his problem? It will take little of his time and effort to find out. And he need not take the advice given him if it does not seem good to him.

Let us suppose, for instance, that Tom proves stubborn in this way. He does not want to go back to being a truck driver; he wants to be his own boss. He feels he got a good start toward being a mechanic in the army, and he has decided to set up an automobile repair shop of his own.

But Ellen is anxious. Suppose he is making a mistake and should fail in the repair business. Their money will be gone, and they will be in debt. In spite of Ellen's anxiety, instead of throwing cold water on Tom's plans and ambitions she seeks the advice of a friend of theirs, a man whose good sense Tom has always admired. The friend talks to Tom and persuades him to hear what the counselor at the Veterans Information Center has to say before he takes any definite steps. After all, he reminds Tom, you don't have to take the advice if you don't want to.

At the Center a counselor takes Tom into his office, offers him a cigarette, and while they light up talks to him a little about his army experience. Tom feels better right away. This guy knows the score; he talks the GI language. Either he's been through the mill himself, or he's talked to a lot of fellows who have. Anyway, he knows what it's all about.

Together they look over Tom's army card, and a chart that the man tells Tom is a picture of his mind and abilities. The few jigsaw lines don't mean anything to Tom, but the counselor can read them as a doctor reads an x-ray. He says they show that Tom has mechanical skill, that he could be a good automobile mechanic all right. He approves of Tom's knowing what he wants to do and tells him his youth and enthusiasm are in his favor. It's good too, he says, that Tom wants to build something for the future.

But he points out from Tom's army record that he has had no actual experience in working on engines, and no training in that part of the mechanic's job. His course of training was never finished in the army. He can repair the chassis, but not the engine.

Tom has to admit this, but says he plans to get that knowledge as he goes along. He thinks that once he has his repair shop he can learn this for himself.

The counselor then reminds him that he will have engines to repair right from the start, and if he does some bad jobs on them while he is trying to learn, he will run the risk of losing the good will and reputation for good work on which his success will depend. Perhaps he would get on all right, but he cannot be sure. And he cannot afford to make a mistake, because he has little money and not much borrowing power at the bank. Wouldn't it be wiser to get a mastery of the automobile repair field before he starts out on his own?

Well, maybe. But how can he get it?

The counselor suggests several ways. Tom might take a job in someone else's repair shop for a while and learn engine repair while he is on the job. If he wants to do this, the counselor will see that the USES finds him such a job. Or why not take advantage of the chance for a year's training in mechanics at the government's expense? If the allowance for living expenses isn't enough, they will get him a part-time job. Or perhaps his wife will want to keep on working for a year. Or if something inside him just insists on being on his own, why not lease a filling station—they will help him find a good one—and take the necessary training in night school?

Thinking hard about possibilities he has not considered before, Tom takes the counselor's suggestions home with him. When he and Ellen have talked them over and chosen among them, he will go back to the counselor at the Center for help in putting into effect the decision he has made. And he will have made it much more wisely than if he had gone ahead without the expert's advice.

If he is physically hurt . . .
HE CAN LIVE AGAIN

Mary and Joe

Older than Ellen by some ten years, Mary, the second of the women waiting on the platform, is also older in experience, in her feelings, and in her thinking. And this is a good thing, because more will be required of Mary than of Ellen. More patience, more self-discipline, more effort in rearranging and readjusting her life. For Mary's husband, Joe, is returning permanently and totally disabled, returning to live the rest of his life in the wheelchair beside which Mary now stands. And the cards that have been dealt Joe are the cards with which Mary too must play the game.

Waiting there on the platform, her hand resting on the shiny wood of the wheelchair, Mary lets her eyes follow a line of telephone poles off into the distance. For the past six months, ever since she learned for sure how badly hurt Joe was and how little improved he could ever be, the sight of telephone poles has at once fascinated and disturbed her. Perhaps because they remind her of the life she and Joe lived before the war, the life she still wants but will not have again.

Joe was a telephone lineman when Mary met him, five years before Pearl Harbor, in a small town where she and her sister ran a beauty shop. Joe had been born and raised on a farm near by.

The most characteristic thing about Joe was his forever wanting action. He always had to be on the go. He didn't finish high school, he used to say, because he couldn't sit still long enough. And wanting action was what took him into the army right off, the second day after Pearl Harbor. No hanging around, no waiting, for him.

Well, he got action all right, Mary thinks bitterly. He got plenty of it right along until he was put out of the fight for good, when an exploding mine demolished the jeep he was riding in and killed three of his buddies instantly. It hadn't killed Joe, but it had used him up pretty badly. When he woke up in a hospital behind the lines he could not move his legs; they were both paralyzed. And for a time he could not speak at all.

Yes, the war has taken a heavy toll of Joe's body. Mary wonders whether it has taken an equal toll of his spirit. Will he still be wanting action? Or will he have lost hope?

From the time he was first wounded, eighteen months ago, through the long stays in one hospital after another, in which doctors and nurses tried to save and restore as much as possible of his body, Mary knows that Joe did not give up, did not lose hope. Six months ago when the army discharged him to the veterans' hospital from which he is coming home today, Mary saw him at the train. Weary, white, and helpless he looked, but he was still full of the old impatience. Even then he was wanting action — wanting the train to get moving so he could get on to the hospital and get well.

How much has he changed, Mary wonders, in these past six months? Does he understand now that doctors can do little more for his body, that they cannot give him back the use of his legs or his ability to speak? Does he realize that they are sending him home at last because they can do no more for him? If so, how is he taking it? Will he be bitter and hard, openly rebellious at his helpless dependence? Or will he be indifferent, despairing, without hope?

Body and mind

Mary is wise to realize that Joe's handicap will be psychological as well as physical. The body and the mind are not separate, independent parts; they are two views of one functioning whole. What happens to one affects the other. When the body is severely injured, the mind is hurt too, and when the mind is sick it may produce serious disorders in the body. Doctors are coming to understand this, to know that they must treat the whole man, not just one part of him. They are being forced to this knowledge by their experience in such cases as this one.

A worker in one of our shipyards lost his right arm in an accident on the job. The wound healed all right, but as the time drew near for the man to leave the hospital, he developed arthritis in his knee. He could not bend it; he could not walk. The joint was red and swollen to three times its normal size, and an x-ray showed an abnormal growth of solid bone all around it.

The standard treatment of the knee had no affect, and the doctor was puzzled—until he discovered the hurt in the man's mind, discovered that he was afraid to leave the hospital because he knew he could no longer hold his old job and didn't know where to find another one. He didn't even know

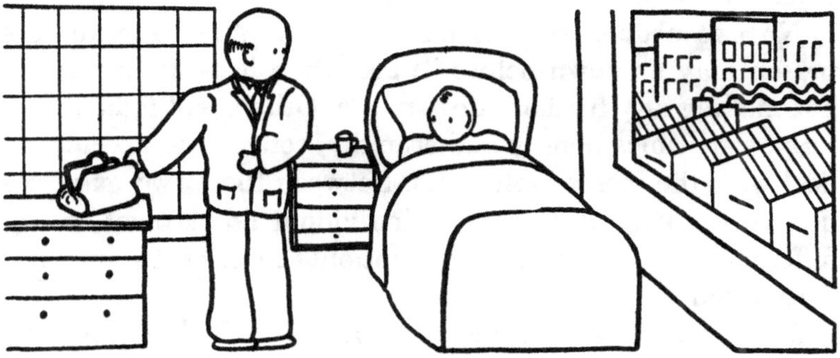

His mind needs doctoring too

what other kind of work he could do without his arm. When the doctor, after a telephone call to the shipyard, was able to tell him that a good job, one he could do easily and well, was waiting for him there, his fear was relieved. The hurt to his mind was healed, and the recovery in his body began at once. In a short time the mass of hard bone around his knee had dissolved, and he was able to leave the hospital.

That story is told by Betsey Barton in her book, *And Now to Live Again*. Miss Barton herself has good reason to know how important are the psychological effects of a physical handicap. An automobile accident some ten years ago left her with a broken back and paralyzed legs, and out of her experience since that time she has come to know that "we are not ever so badly handicapped in our bodies as in our minds. It is our minds that become inflexible and set. It is our minds that lose hope, that feel failure, that shrink from new things and hide away and refuse to come out."

The biggest handicap in any injury is the loss of heart that makes a man say, "What's the use? I can't go on. I'm finished." This is true of any disability, whether it is as permanent and crippling as Joe's and as total blindness or deafness, or a partial disability, such as the loss of an arm or a leg, a bad speech defect, or a disfigurement of the face. Much of what follows in this chapter applies to any handicapped person.

Each in his own way

No two people react to disaster alike. At one extreme a person may lie down before it, accepting it as an excuse for not making any further effort in life. Others will fight it bitterly, sometimes blindly and stupidly, refusing to accept and deal with the inescapable facts. Between these two extremes lie many different degrees of individual adjustment, many different sorts of mental and emotional reaction to hurt and frustration.

For example, at the end of World War I three men, all twenty years old, started out in civilian life with seemingly the same handicap, the loss of both legs. But fifteen years later they were far apart. One was a pencil seller, a beggar, on the streets of a large city. Day in and day out, through rain and snow, he sat on his corner begging, waiting for some in the busy, indifferent, hurrying crowd to stop and drop him a coin.

The second man had become a jeweler. Making his way through the world, he stood not more than four feet high, for he had never bothered to equip himself with artificial legs. At the shop he had a special stool that raised him to the height of his workbench, and here he talked and joked and was as interested in the affairs of the world as those about him. His work was good and nobody in the shop ever stopped to think that he was different from others.

The third man, who learned to use artificial legs skillfully, had become a highly paid business executive. Few of the people he met or worked with ever knew that he was handicapped in any way. On his desk were buttons to push when he wanted something done, and these brought people hurrying to do for him what he would not have done for himself even if he had had his own legs.

It is clear that varying skills, abilities, and interests helped to place these men in such different positions, but the emotional attitude each had toward his handicap was of equal importance in determining the success or failure of their lives.

How a person reacts to disaster depends pretty much on the kind of person he was before, the type of character he had before he was hurt. The sudden crippling of the body does not immediately or of itself make a weak person strong or a strong man weak. There are professional charity-seekers among the handicapped because there are shiftless, lazy people among the able-bodied. The man who became a pencil seller, exhibiting and dramatizing his disability in order to win an easy living from the ready sympathy of others, might have found or imagined some other reason for thinking the world owed him a living even if he had not lost his legs.

This clinging to the established pattern of attitude and reaction is by no means inevitable, however. Human beings can learn new ways of feeling, new ways of tackling problems, of facing life's blows, just as they can learn new skills and develop new interests. Such learning is not easy, but it is possible.

In some cases, of course, the lesser, weaker way is taken through ignorance, because the person himself does not know, and no one tells him, that he does not have to sell pencils or shoelaces. No one tells him that other ways of making a living are open to him, ways that will give him greater happiness and freedom, greater success.

Like the shipyard worker who developed arthritis in his

knee, such a person may want to work, may want to be independent again, but sees no way open to him, and so he becomes afraid and grabs at the first possibility that occurs to him. He needs someone who is better informed, someone who can see more clearly than he, to show him what better ways are possible.

Useful work and enjoyable recreation are possible for almost every handicapped person. But he must discover them and make the necessary effort to learn the new skills they require. The only handicap, according to one expert, that cannot be overcome in some degree is a wooden head.

There is no going back

The ideal reaction to disaster is the attitude put into words by Sir Philip Snowden, the British statesman. When his legs were paralyzed as the result of an accident, at first he did not think the consequences would be permanent, but when, after a long time, he had recovered enough to walk laboriously with the aid of a stout stick, he realized that he would never fully regain the use of his legs. "And it is strange but true," he wrote, "that this conviction brought neither disappointment nor despondency. I calmly reconciled myself to what could not be helped. . . . This has been my philosophy of life. Try to shape circumstances; but if circumstances are too strong to be altered, then accept them with resignation and shape your actions and your conduct according to unalterable fate."

To some this reaction comes as naturally as it apparently did to Sir Philip; it is part of their temperament to approach life "marching breast forward, never doubting clouds will lift." These are the Charles Steinmetz', the Helen Kellers, the Franklin Roosevelts. But for most of us such an attitude must be slowly developed in a constant struggle against our tendency to despair or to waste our time and energies in futile lament.

The chances are that Mary will face this sort of struggle with Joe. Physical activity has been the mainspring of his life and he will not easily accept a role of seemingly helpless inaction. The present and the future will seem hopeless, utterly black. He will wish to God he had shared the fate of his three buddies and will curse the senselessness of things that has brought him to this pass. He will ask—of himself if not of others—the unanswerable question: Why did this happen to me? Why? Why?

And who can blame him?

Perhaps he will have got through the worst of this phase in the hospital, for doctors in army, navy, and veterans' hospitals do their best to pull their patients through it before they are discharged. But if they have not succeeded with Joe, Mary's first and probably most difficult task will be to guide him through to a calmer, more fruitful attitude.

If she is wise she will not play Pollyanna. She will not search frantically for the silver lining to Joe's cloud. There isn't any, and he knows it. She will talk and cry, even curse if necessary, with him for a time. And this will not be hard for her, because she too has plenty of cause for crying and feeling bitter. But after a reasonable time, when they have worked through some of the grief, hurt, and despair, she will bring their mutual consolation to an end, for it can no longer do them any good.

Consider the story of Michael Dowling. As a boy of fourteen he was herding cattle on the northwestern plains. Lost on the Minnesota prairie in a blizzard one night, he stumbled onto a woodpile, which told him that a cabin must be somewhere near. He gathered an armful of the sticks and pivoting slowly in a circle, threw them one after another as far as he could, hoping to locate the shelter. But no sound came back from any of them.

When morning came Michael's hands and feet were frozen stiff. He could see the cabin now and he crawled to its door. Only two feet away lay one of the sticks he had thrown in the night.

When both his legs, his left arm, and all but a stump of the right hand had been amputated, Michael knew the black despair of the newly maimed. He cursed the very vitality that had let him live, that had pulled him through the ordeal of the operation. And again and again he writhed in his bed in a sweat at the thought of that narrow margin of two feet. Why in the name of God had the stick fallen just two feet short? Why? Why?

To ask the question, to search for an answer even when one knows there is no answer, is only human. But it will not change the facts. For Michael it could not change the fateful fall of the wood. If he had continued this futile questioning, he would have become an object of charity for the rest of his life. Instead he turned his back on the past. Taking stock of what was left to him, he decided, to use his own words, that since he'd lost some of the wires down below he must concentrate on improving the power plant in his coconut. So he battled his way through to a normal, happy life, successful far beyond the average.

The point here is a very practical one: However natural the despair, however justified the bitterness, they are futile. They will do no good. So it is up to Mary to get tough with herself and perhaps with Joe. Together they must face the facts of Joe's handicap. They must accept the limitations these facts impose, and then build the best life possible out of what is left to them. What is gone cannot be restored. There is no going back and there is no standing still. There is only forward.

Left to its own devices, the mind has a way of lingering in the past or of slipping off into dreams of miracles in the future, in order to escape the pain of the present. A crippled or disfigured person does not willingly or easily accept the fact that although his legs are gone, his head and his hands remain to be used as he will, or that although sight is lost, hearing and fingertips are left to take over. Instead he will go back, forever and ever back, or forward into fantasy to find some more ideal state than the unpleasant one in which he is.

To want to be at a better starting place, to look and search

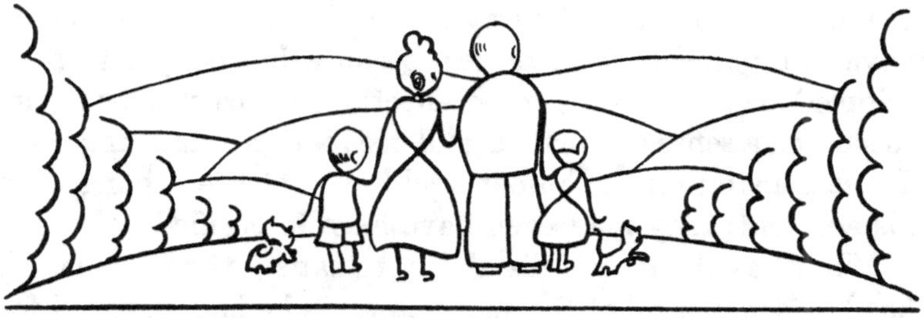

There is only forward

forever for it, is very human, but from the practical point of view it is as silly as the Irishman's reply when the passing Englishman asked him the way to Roscommon.

"Is it to Roscommon you want to go?"

"Yes. That's why I asked you the way."

"Well," said the Irishman, "if I wanted to go to Roscommon, I wouldn't be starting from here."

Probably most of us feel sure that the road to our goal of happiness and usefulness would be easier and shorter if only we could start from some other place. But each person, whatever his handicap—and we all have one or more of some kind—must start the journey from where he stands.

More than meets the eye

The family and friends cannot help the disabled veteran to achieve this forward-looking attitude without understanding something of his feelings and his problems. They can never wholly share his state of mind, but they can try, if they will, to imagine how things seem to him. They can try to experience enough of his fears and his hurt to understand rather than condemn his actions. It is a sound policy that requires workers with the blind at the Seeing Eye school in New Jersey to live for a month with their eyes tightly bandaged all the time, before they begin to teach those who are without sight.

Proper understanding might begin with the fundamental fact that the psychological or inner needs of the handicapped person are still those of every human being. His basic needs have not vanished or lessened because his body has been crippled. He still needs love, affection, security, friendship, social life, a sense of worth, useful occupation, refreshing play. These demands of the human soul have not been changed by his accident; they may even have been intensified.

What has changed is his ability to satisfy these needs. He has lost some or all of the specific means he had acquired for fulfilling them, and if he is to regain happiness, if he is to live again, he must acquire a set of substitute satisfactions. If he can no longer dance, play tennis, dive, and swim with his friends, he must learn to take pleasure in beating them at chess, checkers, or a rousing game of poker, in the vicarious excitement of the armchair sports expert, or perhaps in a totally new interest such as music or reading.

This will, of course, not prove as simple as it sounds. Psychological needs do not make themselves known so recognizably as the physical need for food, for instance, and the individual may not be aware of their presence, so that he does not know what is wrong with him or what he should do about it. And even if he does recognize and admit these needs, the newly handicapped person may shrink from even the first steps toward satisfying them.

He may, for example, long for the companionship of his family, yet not want to leave the hospital and return to them. And they will be puzzled, bewildered, perhaps even hurt by his behavior. There is a room ready for him, one more comfortable than his hospital room. And the surroundings at home are much pleasanter than the gray and white of the hospital. His family, his friends are all waiting to receive him back with open arms. The fact that he is missing some parts of his body does not change their feeling for him. Why should he feel uneasy or refuse to come home?

Let them look at the matter from his point of view. In his first weakness, his first comprehension of the frightful thing that has happened to him, he has found a haven in the hospital. Helpless and sick, he has been scarcely conscious of the presence of the doctors and nurses. He has got used to them. He no longer minds their seeing his deformity or disfigurement. He has got used, too, to the hospital world and the comfortable monotony of its routine. Its demands upon him are not more than he can meet; its tomorrow is not of his planning.

But home? Home is an unfamiliar and fearful world. To you, it is the same house, the same room, the same furniture. But to him it is strange, a world in which he has never lived — because he has never lived in any world without sight or legs or arms, whichever the case may be. And so he shrinks from facing it and all its strangeness. He has no incentive or energy to meet its problems and demands. He may shrink too from close contact with those he loves best, for they are strangers to his helplessness or his disfigurement.

An American paratrooper, straight and six-foot-two when he left his wife and six-year-old son, returned from a mission over Holland with his chest shattered and his back broken. When the doctors and nurses had made him as well as they could and he was discharged from the hospital, he refused to go home. All bent over now like a five-foot question mark, he could not face his little son. "What'd he think of his old man now?" he asked.

So he was sent to a convalescent home in New York City, a home where special attention was being given to such cases of mental hurt. As if by coincidence, a couple of six-year-olds in the neighborhood were in and out of the house a dozen times a day. They pestered the ex-paratrooper to play with them, to fly their model airplanes, to tell them about the real planes and the fighting he had seen. At the end of a week, he said to the doctor in charge, "I guess I'll go home now." And he went.

Once the injured man is at home, however, his fears are likely to extend to the wider world of business and social relationships in which he was formerly quite at ease. He may want to hide away in a back bedroom, refusing to see visitors or to meet anyone outside the family. He is lonely, lonelier than he has ever been. He wants, and needs, the companionship of friends, the release and stimulation of good times with other people. But he dreads too much the thought of their eyes upon his disfigured face, his withered or missing arm, his twisted or useless legs.

Most of us have experienced in some degree the unpleasant paralysis of self-consciousness, and many able-bodied individuals find it difficult, in some cases almost impossible, to meet strangers or to walk into a room full of people, even of people they know. Imagine then the feelings of the disfigured or the crippled, who have many times more reason for shrinking from what seems such an ordeal.

Understanding this feeling in the handicapped person, appreciating its strength and depth, is helpful; giving in to it is not. In most cases self-consciousness of any sort is based upon an exaggeration of one's defects, real or imagined, and of their effect on other people. For instance, few of us pay any attention, beyond perhaps a casual first notice, to the tiny contrivance worn nowadays to improve one's hearing. Yet those who work with the deafened say that the biggest obstacle in helping these persons is their vanity—their extreme unwillingness to wear hearing aids. And men, they say, are worse in this respect than women!

Much of the difficulty, the exaggeration of the defect, comes from too much thinking about one's self. The authors of *Normal Lives for the Disabled* tell the story of a crippled girl, now a governor's secretary, who started her comeback in the workaday world in the business office of a small inn in a college community. She knew that she was supposed to take her meals in the dining room with the guests, but she chose instead to eat in the kitchen with the hired help.

At the end of a week, her employer asked for an explanation of this behavior, and she explained that she did not wish to inflict the sight of her badly crippled body upon the guests. The man's answer was rough but straight. "Part of your job is to be pleasant to the guests at dinner. If you enter that dining room with your mind interested in the guests instead of on your body, you will draw their attention to what is on your mind and not to your body. At any rate, that's the job; take it or leave it."

She took it, and it headed her up the road to success. She had thought she was an eyesore and that everyone else would think so too. Since her employer evidently did not think so, her job was to learn how not to be one, and in her own words, "It's not hocus-pocus. It's just a fact—that when I really stopped thinking about my body, other people did too."

There is no Santa Claus

There is no magic that will produce the new life for the handicapped, no short cut to it. There is no Santa Claus to bring it in his pack and deposit it beside the chimney complete and ready for use. Neither the new skills nor the new mental habits that are needed spring into being overnight; learning them is a *process,* a slow and difficult process, especially in the beginning. It will take patience, courage, and unwearying determination on the part of the individual himself and in his family as well.

But here again the longest journey begins with a single step. And the person, whatever handicap he has to overcome, must begin with the things he *can* do, no matter how little or seemingly useless they may be. Then gradually widen his circle of activities, calling for a little more effort, a little longer reach, from day to day. Increase by slow degrees the number of things he does for himself; lessen slowly but firmly the area of his dependence on others.

Remember that his strongest need is for self-confidence, for faith in his ability to do what he must do, for belief that he can learn what he must learn.

Words alone are seldom enough to give his morale the boost it needs. Sermons and exhortations will not develop the courage and patience he must have. For this there must be *works* too, things he can do and in which he can eventually see and feel a measure of success. But at first he may have to rely on the faith and courage of others—his doctor, his wife, his mother.

One man whose arm was paralyzed as the result of a series of operations was told to stand along the wall, touching it with his finger and trying each time to raise the finger a fraction of an inch above the mark he had reached the time before. This seemed very silly to him, and hopeless. He could see no returns from his efforts, and he despaired a hundred times a day. He could never recover the use of his arm.

It took constant encouragement from others to keep him at the exercise. It took constant assurance that this effort was worth while and would produce results. After a while he himself could see evidence of improvement, could see the finger marks climbing on the wall, could feel his arm a little freer in motion. Then his own faith, his own courage, his own patience took over the task of making him persevere.

Betsey Barton's first steps on the road back were even less certain. After years of hospitals, doctors, operations, and treatments, she was still flat on her back in bed, to all appearances completely helpless. Then to her bedside came a wise man. "There are two things you can do," he told her. "You can breathe. So breathe, like this." And he showed her how. "And you can move your stomach muscles. So move them, like this." And he showed her how.

What good would that do? Miss Barton wondered. The man explained. "You needn't believe this," he told her. "Just do these things, as I have shown you, and you will see what good they do."

So Miss Barton breathed and moved her stomach muscles as she had been told, blindly trusting at first, until she could feel the results within herself. Then, with a hope and a determination she had thought never to feel again, she was ready for the next step. Today she walks, on crutches and in braces to be sure, but she walks. She gets all around New York City on her own. She travels across the continent. She writes. But her recovery of independence began with those two things: breathing and moving her stomach muscles.

One must take careful thought in urging a handicapped person to efforts on his own behalf. He must not be pushed too far or too fast. The tasks must not be beyond his present powers, must not exceed his endurance or capacity for effort. For if too much is asked of him when he is already weak and of little faith, he will fail in his attempt and the end will be worse than the beginning. It will be harder, much harder, for him to try again. Too many failures will destroy his will to try; they will make him more hopeless than before.

The better way

It is a distressing paradox that the person who loves another the most may prove the most persistent enemy in his battle for independence. A striking illustration of this is given in Katharine Butler Hathaway's story of her life, *The Little Locksmith*. Stunted by a disease of the spine when she was a youngster, Katharine never grew taller than a ten-year-old child. Yet within her small body lived a passionate, free spirit that demanded independence and sought it in writing. Each day she would lock herself alone in her room and write for two or three hours. These were her happiest times, for in them she was whole, no longer bound by her misshapen body

But Katharine's mother often spoiled these hours for her. She would be waiting in the hall outside when Katharine came from her room, waiting with anxious questions. Why had she been so long? Why did she shut herself away like that? What was it she wanted that her mother wasn't giving her?

When Katharine tried to explain what these hours of freedom did for her, Mrs. Butler would say sadly, "You don't love me. I can't seem to make you happy."

And Katharine would answer passionately, "I do love you, very much. But I don't want you to *make* me happy. I *am* happy, in myself. I am the happiest person in the world at times."

It is easy to see what was wrong. Mrs. Butler was smothering Katharine with her love; her emotions had got out of hand. For years the care of Katharine had been her sole concern. Her heart aching with grief and pity for the girl's handicap, she felt she couldn't do enough for her. She wanted to protect her from the world, shield her against hurt and suffering, make her path as smooth and easy as it could be. The very intensity and singleness of her love blinded her to the fact that in seeking to wrap Katharine in cotton wool she was defeating her own dearest desire: her daughter's happiness.

Love that is truly wise may often appear harsh and cruel. It will refuse to show its pity, to be sentimental, or to coddle. The wise mother or wife will, however hard it is for her, refuse to do anything for the handicapped son or husband that he can do for himself. It may wring her heart with pity to watch his fumbling, laborious efforts to tie his own shoelaces or cut his own meat. She could do it for him so easily, and save him such painful, embarrassing trouble. But she will not do it.

Nor will she give all her time to fussing over him, to keeping him occupied and amused. He must learn to live as fully as possible on his own resources. He may resent it at the time, may even call her hard-hearted. And so may other people whose pity is greater than their wisdom. But in the end it will mean greater happiness for him as well as for her.

In training blind people to use guide dogs, it is part of the philosophy at Seeing Eye that no one can *give* a man his independence; he must find it for himself. So once new pupils have been told where to hang their clothes, where to find the dining room, the bathroom, the recreation room, they are expected to find these places for themselves. If they lose a sock or a shoe, they may ask someone to help them find it only after they have made a thorough search of their own. They are expected to butter their own bread, cut their own meat. If they complain that they have never done these things for themselves, they are told it is high time they started.

The same attitude prevails in the re-education given at the

Institute for the Crippled and Disabled in New York City. There the people must learn not only to walk with braces and crutches or canes, but to walk with them on slippery, highly polished floors. When someone falls down, no one rushes to pick him up. More likely everybody laughs.

Cruel? No, for by this method the person learns to get up by himself and also soon gets over his terrifying embarrassment at falling. The Institute's aim is to force the handicapped to cope with situations which they will have to meet in the normal world of competition and business, the world of hurrying people, of revolving doors, of waxed floors.

But — and this is very important — they are not forced to deal with these situations until they are ready for them. They are not left to get up from a fall by themselves if it is physically impossible for them to do so. They are not left alone in a chair in the middle of an empty room unless it is physically possible for them to get out of that chair and across to the door alone. They are not left to find their way without help down the hall and through the heavy door to the taxi that has been called for them until they are physically able to do so.

Experience has shown the Institute workers, however, that a person is almost always able to do these things before he himself feels that he is ready for them. Usually he must be urged and pushed a little farther than he thinks he can go.

Some do's and don'ts

Take the trouble to be informed about his handicap and the best ways of dealing with it. It is too bad that there is not in every community a good re-education center like the Institute for the Crippled and Disabled in New York City. A center where the newly disabled could learn, in company with others equally handicapped or more so, the most effective and least tiring ways of handling his new body, could be fitted with the proper and most useful mechanical or artificial aids, and could learn how to manage them skillfully. A center where he could be taught, or at least shown, the attitudes and approaches most likely to get him over the highest hurdles in his readjustment to life.

Perhaps someday such centers will be an accepted part of our social welfare program. In the meantime the family of a man returning disabled should be in touch with the nearest rehabilitation agency, so as to profit as fully as possible from the guidance and advice those with training and experience can give. If you do not know the best agency in your community, ask the Veterans Service Committee or the Red Cross.

Or you may write for information to the Federal Office of Vocational Rehabilitation (Washington 25, D.C.), or to any one of the following national organizations: the Institute for the Crippled and Disabled (400 First Avenue, New York City), the American Foundation for the Blind (15 West Sixteenth Street, New York City), the American Society for the Hard of Hearing (1537 Thirty-fifth Street N.W., Washington, D.C.), the National Tuberculosis Association (1790 Broadway, New York City), or the American Heart Association (1790 Broadway, New York City). These organizations will be glad to give you information about the kinds of work done by people with handicaps in particular fields, or to help you in any way they can.

Give him time. If the soldier coming home normal and unimpaired lives for a time in another world of values, so that we find it difficult to communicate with him because we do not speak the same language, how much more so the man with the added handicap of a physical disability. You must expect him to be lethargic, apathetic, indifferent, depressed, lazy—for a time. Do not goad and scold. Instead, concentrate on getting him interested and busy in spite of himself.

Treat him as a person, not as a cripple. His body may be different, but the chances are that his character and personality are the same as before. And the physical difference of which he is so conscious will make him want all the more to be the normal human being he was before he went away. So treat him like one. Do not set him apart. Try to decrease rather than increase his sense of being a fractional man.

Help him to feel that society values him as an individual—not only as a hero who has made an important contribution to the nation's welfare, but as an individual who is accepted and liked for his own sake, because his company is enjoyable. According to psychologists, a real and sincere concern for the individual and his problems will count more toward his rehabilitation than all the most complicated and special techniques.

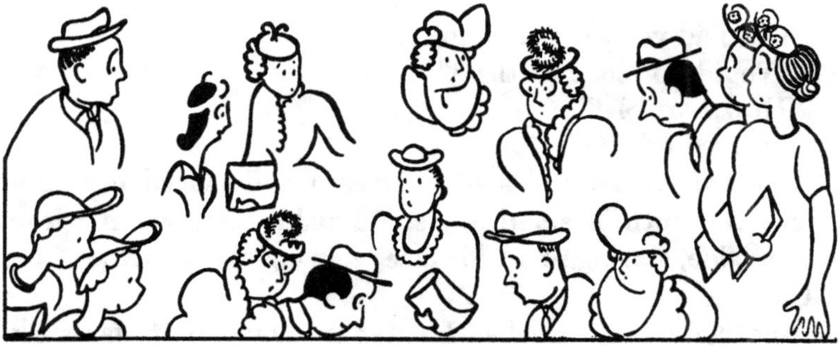

Turn those eyes away

The OWI has given some sound advice in this connection: "If you are disturbed by the disfigurement or deformity, discipline yourself so that your disturbance is not apparent. Do not let horror or sorrow appear on your face or in your voice or manner. It is up to you to make him realize . . . that you feel about him exactly as always, and that his disfigurement is unimportant compared with your affection or friendship."

Above all—and this is particularly applicable to friends, acquaintances, or strangers on the street—do not stare. Do not fix your eyes in curiosity on an artificial hand, a twisted face, a glass eye.

In the February 24, 1945, issue of the *Saturday Evening Post,* Lieutenant Marshall Davenport, who lost a leg and was badly burned in a tank in North Africa and after a year in a German prison camp was returned to this country, tells how he has had to fight his hardest battle against the thoughtlessness of his countrymen.

While still undergoing plastic surgery he left the hospital one afternoon for his first walk. After the barbed wire of the prison camp, the thrill of being free to walk through the hospital gates was so great that he walked in and out several times. "Look, no guard, no guard," he kept repeating.

But he had not gone far until he was wishing he was back in the hospital, back even in the prison camp — anyplace to be off the street and away from the stares and remarks of the passers-by.

"Oh! Did you see that soldier!"

"Would you look at that!"

"How horrible!"

"Scarred for life!"

One woman let out a little scream and placed her hand over her mouth. A small boy stood at his feet, walking from side to side, staring up at his face, viewing the wreckage from all sides.

Another afternoon when Lieutenant Davenport was walking along the street the waist strap broke on his artificial leg. He tried holding the leg in place with his hand, but the broken strap dragged out the end of his trouser leg so that it was impossible to walk. He had to stop, roll up his pants leg, and remove the broken strap. And he had to play this scene before the largest audience he had ever had.

It may be natural for people who have not been touched by calamity to be curious about those who have, but they should seek better ways of satisfying this curiosity than staring and asking thoughtless questions.

In Lieutenant Davenport's words: "Beneath the surface of that war-torn veteran whom you see on the street, there is a man. . . . He asks no favors, no sympathy, and no special consideration. He asks only that he be treated with the same courtesy and respect that are due any other civilized human being. He asks only for a fair chance."

Don't be a "cheer-up guy." This is a handicapped man's own phrase, and he speaks it with scorn, for the over-cheery friends who come around telling him to buck up, he isn't so bad off, he might be a lot worse, and so on. In the words of the OWI again, "The man you are visiting may feel depressed. It is his right to feel so. It is an offense to his dignity and his common sense to go into a routine of transparent 'cheeriness.' The express intent of cheering up is seldom convincing or beneficial to minimize the crippling effect of maiming. By facing the reality of a man's disability yourself, you can help him face it."

Lend him an ear, but do not pry. Be natural and casual in your conversation. Don't ask a lot of questions or give unsought advice. If the man wants to talk about his disability, how he got it and what he's going to do about it, listen with interest, understanding, and sympathy—not with pity. Don't flood him with a lot of observations and opinions! But if he does not wish to talk, don't pester him with questions just to satisfy your own curiosity. Respect his wishes.

Strange as it seems, this needs to be said to people who are not close to the handicapped person, who do not even know him. Lieutenant Davenport says that almost every day some stranger comes up and asks, "How'd you get it, soldier?"

"Oh, my poor boy. How did it happen?" an old lady passing on the street asks a soldier whose face is badly scarred.

"I don't mean to get personal, soldier, but do you mind telling me how it happened? Where did you lose it?" a man in a bar or restaurant asks the soldier who is missing an arm or a leg.

"What is that? What does it mean?" the bright young thing asks the wearer of the Purple Heart.

Lieutenant Davenport's answer is simply, "I was burned in a tank." But it takes a lot of control not to tell the stranger to mind his own business.

That people who ask such questions mean well there is little doubt. And the soldiers realize this, even the ones who shut them up with smart answers. They understand that people want to help but don't know what to do, that they ask these questions in good faith and with sincerity. "But if they really want to help us," the soldiers say, "why don't they let us alone?"

Do not ignore his handicap. It seems to be the present tendency to advise families to greet their disabled men casually, without emotion, but Willard Waller applies sounder psychology when he qualifies this advice in *The Veteran Comes Back*: "Do not start being hard-boiled until you have been sympathetic."

At first the handicap is, naturally and inevitably, the most important thing in the world for both the man and his family. Their minds are full of it. How unnatural, then, for them to ignore it in conversation, to refuse to mention it. The silent treatment will only make it grow bigger and bigger in their thoughts, instead of smaller and smaller as it should.

No good purpose is served by pretending the disfigurement or disability does not exist. It's there all right, a cold, hard fact that must be reckoned with. And since both the man and his family must reckon with it, the best and most natural way is to bring it out into the open, to talk about it, cry about it. Giving way for a time to the pain and grief you all feel is better than locking them up within you, to fester and ferment into nervous tensions and mental complexes.

After this it will be time enough to be brave, to concentrate on what is left instead of what is gone, to reassemble the pieces in the best life possible. But even then, when the disaster has receded into its proper place in the past, it must not be allowed to become a horrible can't-ever-be-mentioned thing. It should always be possible to refer to it naturally when necessary. For only then can you be sure you are seeing it in its proper perspective, that your attitude toward it is a healthy one.

Give him love and affection but not pity. In the flood of your own emotion about his plight, you are likely to err on the side of love, giving him too much when too little would be better for him. Unable to control your own tenderness you will seek to express it by having him lean on you. You will tend to forget that what he needs, whether he knows it or not, is to stand on his own two feet, even if they're wooden ones or encased in metal. This is the time to get hard-boiled if necessary — but first with yourself.

Don't help him unless he asks for help — and not always then. Don't wait on him too much. It is a very significant fact that handicapped children from poor homes usually make better progress toward independence than those from wealthier families. When circumstances force the handicapped individual to fend for himself if he is to eat and to be comfortable, he will more quickly and readily achieve self-reliance. The wealthy child knows he will not go hungry, will not be without a place to sleep, and his inner need for independence must be very strong to overcome this unconscious knowledge that someone else will take care of him if he does not make the effort to take care of himself.

Everybody wants to help, of course, but very often their good intentions produce harmful results. For instance, a person who has learned to walk in braces has probably had to achieve, by laborious effort, a very precise and delicate sense of coordination and timing. When he gets up from a chair or steps from a curbstone or into an automobile, there is a stage or two in the process when his balance is very precarious. If at this moment some anxious and well-meaning friend or some let-me-help-you-up stranger grabs him by the arm, the result may be anything but help, may even prove disastrous. A much better way is to offer your help and let the person tell you what, if anything, he wants you to do.

Here is another instance: A blind man, obviously coming from work since he carried a lunch box, got on a streetcar. There was no vacant seat, so he stood just inside the door, with his back to the money box. Some high school boys near by noticed him but did not offer him their seats. Seeing this, a man sitting some distance away glared hard at the boys and his lips got tighter and tighter. It was clear that he was thinking hard thoughts about the younger generation.

At last he could stand it no longer. Rising from his seat, he went back to the blind man, took him by the arm, and drew him along the aisle to the vacant seat. "But I'm just going a few blocks," the blind man protested. It was no use. The kind man, realizing his blessings and this poor man's lack of them, saw to it that the blind man sat. So three or four blocks farther on, the blind man had to find his way through a crowded aisle to the end of the car.

It is obvious that this stranger was a kind man. So kind that he could not bear to sit while another less fortunate than he stood up. And he would have been very shocked indeed had anyone told him that instead of helping the blind man he had given him a good hard kick. The blind man was getting on all right, and was undoubtedly happy to know that he could hold a useful job and could travel to and from work on the streetcar, handling himself quite competently in the homeward rush. In the face of such hard-earned independence, the stranger's play of pity must have been a bruising kick.

Handicapped people very often do need help from strangers. This same blind man, when he came to get off the streetcar, knew that he needed help in crossing to the curb in front of oncoming automobiles. And he asked for it. He simply laid his hand on the shoulder of the person in front of him, who looked around and took in the situation at a glance. He tucked the blind man's arm firmly under his, and with a casual "Well, we're getting the cold wave they promised us, aren't we?" walked with him to the sidewalk. Then he went on his way with a cheery "Good night. I go straight ahead and I see you turn to the left."

In this case the man's kindness was of real help. He waited until he was asked and then he did neither more nor less than was wanted, and did it without ceremony, confusion, or comment. Such treatment allows the handicapped man to live in his own way, sure of a helping hand when he needs it but not made conspicuous by help that he does not want or need.

Plan for the future intelligently and carefully, so that it will not be a barren life of invalidism, a sterile life of incapacity. For this no amount of money or care will compensate. As Tagore has said, "He who weeps when he misses the sun may also miss the stars." There might be some point in missing the stars if by doing so you could regain the sun. But you can't. So build a future upon what is left, not upon what is gone. Take a lesson in practical wisdom from this little verse:

> As you travel on through life, Brother,
> Whatever be your goal,
> Keep your eye upon the doughnut
> And not upon the hole.

In planning the new interests that are to be developed, the new skills to be learned, take careful stock of the training, experience, and abilities of your serviceman so that the plan will not be beyond his powers. To make a successful adjustment to his handicap does not mean that he should try to become a Franklin Roosevelt or a Philip Snowden; few persons even with whole bodies achieve their stature. Keep the goals within the realm of what is possible. If he always had trouble with arithmetic in school, don't urge him to try bookkeeping.

On the other hand, do not reject an occupation or skill just because he's never thought of it or done that sort of thing before. He undoubtedly has hidden talents and interests that he has never discovered. In uncovering these and developing them lies his greatest chance for a happy life. His enforced leisure may permit him to try his hand at something he has always wanted to do but could not find time for. Skulda Banér could never find time to write the stories that crowded her mind when she was earning her living in an advertising agency. But when glaucoma took away her sight, these stories and her ability to type became her key to continued usefulness and happiness. She is now well on the way to achieving recognition as an American writer.

The plan for the future must include your life as well as his. Make sure that it includes some outside interests, some activities that do not center on him and his problems. If he is completely helpless and you cannot afford to hire an attendant for him, this may seem almost impossible. But do not hesitate to call on your friends to stay with him if he cannot be left alone. Most of them will be glad to be shown some way in which they can help you. And a few hours away several days a week will make you much better company for him and for yourself the rest of the time.

Don't let him slump into passive, lonely gloom. By all means require of him some social and recreational activities. All work and no play is as bad for the handicapped as for the able-bodied. He should develop such hobbies as his condition permits. Stamp collecting, singing, reading, carpentry, radio, the movies — all or most such activities will be possible for him as recreational diversions to supplement good times with friends.

You will realize, though perhaps he will not at present, that friendship is not based on physical appearance. Once people, old friends and new, have got used to his handicap, they will hardly be aware of it. It is he, not his body, they will like or dislike; it is his mind, his spirit, his personality that will make them want his company or avoid it.

Here a word to the friends is in order. Take thought for the ease and comfort of the handicapped person you are entertaining in your home. Take the time to find out what special arrangements will help him, then make them. Push those odd little tables out of the way of his crutches or wheelchair — *before he arrives*. Take your blind friend around your house and show him where things are, show him how to use the radio and the phonograph. But don't tell him the davenport is "over there"; tell him it is "two steps forward and one to the left." See that he has a good sharp knife for cutting his meat, and learn how to arrange his plate in the accepted manner for the blind. It goes clockwise: the meat at twelve, potato at three, vegetables at six, and relish at nine. The water stands at the right, bread and butter to the left.

Arrange for him to spend some of his time — not all of it — with other handicapped persons. Being with others who have been as badly hurt has a healing value. It will show him what others have done and can do, and to know something *can* be done gives him confidence. It may not make the *doing* any easier, but it will keep him trying. It will show him that his handicap and his problems are not unique.

This is the principle behind the treatment prescribed for some deafened men in army hospitals. To their bedsides come pretty girls who talk with them, writing questions and comments on pads of paper. After several such conversations, the girls reveal the fact that they too are deaf. The surprised men, knowing that the girls have had no trouble understanding them, realize that they too can learn to read lips successfully and inconspicuously.

Books about people who have succeeded in overcoming a major handicap are helpful too. But words, however right and wise, will not carry the same weight as seeing and talking with someone who has successfully dealt with a handicap. The "buddy" system used by the AAF recognizes this therapeutic value of working with others in a like predicament. When a man enters a rehabilitation center he is assigned a buddy with whom he does his exercises in the gym and who helps him keep a record of his progress. In the hospital a man with a broken leg is paired with a man who has a broken arm, so each can help the other with the particular exercises he cannot manage. This keeps the man from getting bored with his own case and from being discouraged about his own progress.

Don't expect too much of him. Remember that physical disability is tiring. This is especially true if the disability involves the manipulation of mechanical contrivances such as artificial limbs or braces, for these greatly complicate the routine activities of everyday life. It takes more time, more energy, for the handicapped person to do the little things an able-bodied person does almost automatically. So allow for this and plan for it in whatever schedule is set up for his day and week.

The future will be what they make it

On some such principles as these, then, Mary and Joe will arrange the pattern of their future. As objectively as possible they will examine Joe's special needs and Mary's, their hopes and dreams, their assets, their liabilities, their likes and dislikes. All these factors in living must be brought together, given a good shake, turned upside down, and the pieces rearranged according to the situation as it now is.

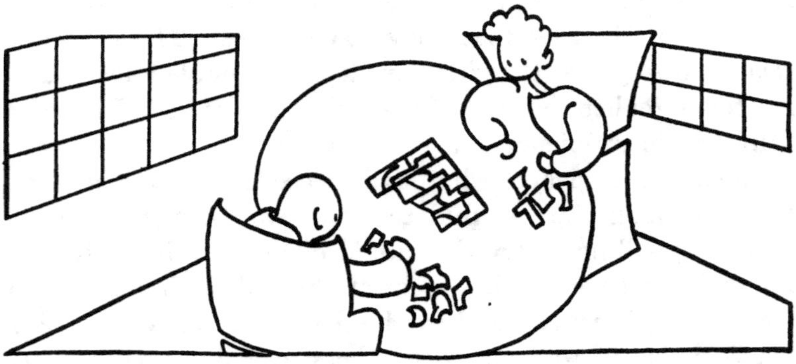

Fit the pieces together

And in this process many purely practical considerations must be taken into account. For instance, from now on steps and stairs will be a major consideration in determining where they live, the houses they visit, the buildings in which they transact business or seek amusement. The number of steps to the front or back door will become more important than the view or the closet space in choosing their house. Or if they prefer an apartment, the absence or presence of an elevator will determine whether they must put up with the street noise on the first floor or can escape it by living on the eighth.

The best for Joe probably would be a first-floor duplex on a level site with plenty of yard space for a garden. Or a small house of his own, a bungalow, with enough room for a garden. There will be no reason why, after a while at least, he cannot wield a hoe and rake from his wheelchair. But ease of passage for his wheelchair will have to replace pure aesthetic considerations in the arrangement of flower beds without and of furniture within. No chairs and tables and desks jutting out in odd places any more. Flat against the wall will be better now.

It will take foresight and ingenuity to arrange convenient transportation for Joe in his chair, but it can be done. They will need to devise a kind of ramp that can be put in place as a runway down a few steps or into the car. It must be wide and heavy enough to hold the wheelchair, yet light enough for Mary to handle. The standard front seat of the car must be removed and a special driver's seat installed that will leave room for Joe's chair and space besides for tucking in the ramp itself. With these arrangements and with Mary to drive, Joe can once more enter the world of motion pictures, plays, concerts, dining out in restaurants and hotels, visiting friends who don't live too high up, picnics and excursions into the country.

He may hate all this at first. The need for these special arrangements will irk him; he won't like being conspicuous; he will hate the commotion his coming always causes. But he will get used to it, and as he and Mary and his friends learn the necessary routine so that it works more smoothly, he will enjoy the wider, richer life it makes possible.

Arrangements for as active a life as possible are especially important for Mary and Joe, because the nature of Joe's particular injury will make further sexual activity impossible for them. This presents a problem not only for Joe but for Mary too. Young and healthy as she is, she will almost certainly face the need for channeling a normal sexual drive into other kinds of outlets.

Fortunately for her prospects of happiness in these circumstances, sexual need is not a purely physical thing. It is bound up with needs for love, tenderness, and companionship, and these phases of it Mary may still have in full measure. Physical satisfaction is perhaps the lesser part of the sexual relationship; people can do without it if necessary without suffering greatly, providing they learn to work off the resultant strain and tension in other activities—in sports, music, an absorbing job, or lively good times, for instance.

The seriousness of the problem this sexual deprivation creates will vary with the individual. If Mary finds it looming too large for her to cope with successfully herself, she will do well to seek skilled help—from a psychiatrist perhaps, or from the psychiatric social worker on the local staff of the Red Cross or the family welfare agency.

A cushion is not enough

Fortunately, Mary and Joe will not have to worry about essential expenses, because Joe will have the monthly pension allowed him for life because of his disability.

Pensions for disabled veterans are based on the extent of the disability as determined by a rating board composed of a doctor, a lawyer, and a vocational expert, who have all the records and findings in the individual case and an established schedule of disability ratings to base their decision on. Information on all matters concerning pensions, rating problems, medical care, and hospitalization can be secured from the Veterans Administration, the officers of one of the service organizations, or the Red Cross. (See pages 35 to 37.)

Joe's pension plus the various other benefits to which he is entitled because of his total and permanent disability will give him and Mary a good financial cushion, but they will be wise not to rest entirely upon it. Their monthly income will be enough to relieve them of worry about food and shelter and essential clothing, but it will not permit the little luxuries, the indulgence in hobbies, the range of recreation and amusements that can add so much to their enjoyment of living. Nor will trying to manage on the pension alone be good for their mental health. From this standpoint they should both have some useful and gainful occupation.

It may not prove practicable for Mary to take a job away from home, but why should she not resume the work she did before she married Joe and have a beauty shop of her own? She might set it up in the front room of the house or down the hallway in the apartment building, in either case within sufficiently easy reach of Joe's wheelchair. This would give Mary an interest of her own and some time away from Joe, thereby forcing him into a degree of independence that otherwise might not come too readily. It would prove one of the best possible safeguards against Mary's taking over the whole of Joe's life for him, against her developing the kind of smothering oversolicitude that proved so painful to Katharine Hathaway.

It is true that taking on the responsibility of a business of her own will require more careful planning from Mary. She will have to budget her time and arrange her schedule to fit the program of things she must do for Joe. Since she is to be his chauffeur, she may have to plan well ahead in order to leave time between shampoos for driving him to the doctor or the lawyer or the tailor or to and from work if he has a job outside. But it will be well worth the cost in effort.

There is no real reason why Joe himself can't do some kind of useful work and contribute to the family pocketbook too, even though such contribution may not be needed. After all, his mind and his hands are as useful as ever. His occupational opportunities out in the labor market are limited of course, but he may be surprised at the chances he will have if he takes stock of his abilities, masters some skill that requires neither walking nor speaking, and with Mary's help tries to find a place. If he can do a necessary job and do it well, he may easily find an employer who will be more than willing to make the necessary arrangements for his wheelchair.

Perhaps the first thing he should do is finish his high school work by correspondence. The sitting still won't bother him now as it did before. Then, if his abilities and interests permit, he might learn to type or to keep books, both very useful skills in the business world.

If this doesn't prove possible, or if Joe prefers some other arrangement, there are many things he might learn to do at home. He might put his experience to use by developing an electrical repair shop. Or he might go in for radio repair, or jewelry-making if he has any artistic bent, or fine woodworking. Acquiring his tools, arranging his workbench or workroom so that it will be convenient for him in his chair, and developing his skill will occupy him for many absorbed hours.

And if he becomes thoroughly skilled in whatever field he chooses, he need not worry about clients and customers; they will seek him out wherever he does his work.

If he has no special interests, or in his discouragement cannot put his finger on them, he can find out what they are by taking some aptitude tests. Someone at the Veterans Information Center or the Veterans Administration office will arrange these for him, and a vocational counselor will help him decide what would be most profitable for him to learn, both in personal satisfaction and in money. The counselor will be able to tell him too what openings he is likely to find in the various crafts, trades, and professions.

Ride a hobby

To the skill he chooses to develop in the hope of earning money, he should add a hobby — or two or three. Hobbies are of great benefit to anyone, but especially to one handicapped like Joe. Whether he substitutes for the tennis he would like to play the vicarious enjoyment of matches and tournaments

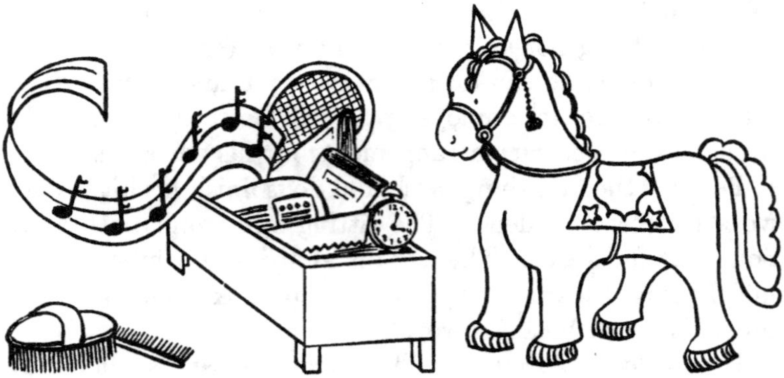

Tend it well and ride it hard

through the sports page or goes in for something quite different, such as photography or music, makes little difference. But he should never be without a hobbyhorse. He should ride it hard, tend and feed it well, and it will carry him far.

One hobby that might please him would be the making

and staging of puppet shows. Just a taste of puppetry might put him under its spell for years. Not only would it give him a direct outlet for the action he craves and for feelings that he cannot ever express in words, but it would be a means of his giving genuine pleasure to his friends.

Or there is the whole realm of domestic accomplishment open to him. He probably left all this to Mary before, but now he might try his hand at plain and fancy cooking and surprise himself by finding satisfaction in turning out tasty soups, stews, and pastries. Many a man has made a hobby of cooking, and it is a truism that the world's best professional cooks are men.

But cook from a wheelchair? Of course, if it is planned for and suitable arrangements are made. Betsey Barton describes her pleasure when once she was left all alone for several days on a western ranch because the companion-maid-cook she had taken with her deserted her in search of a more agreeable climate. While she waited for a less temperamental aide to be found, she learned to make beds from her wheelchair and to mop the floors, clean enough. And she learned to cook. "I shall never forget the day I put all the things in the kitchen where I could reach them, in bottom shelves and drawers. No one coming in then could ever find anything, and I refused to show them."

One hunting enthusiast, in spite of his wheelchair, has not missed a single season for the past ten years. He buys a license and goes to the hunting lodge with friends. He enjoys their company, and he stays at the lodge while they are shooting. He says he gets as much kick out of this, except for missing the exercise, as he did when he actually shot the game himself.

In all this process of adjustment, Mary and Joe will have to make a nice discrimination between a legitimate hope for improvement in Joe's condition and a fruitless search for some miracle-worker to bring it about. Although good doctors have told them that no more can be done for Joe now, this does not necessarily mean that no way of making him better will ever be found. Certainly not at the present rate of advance in medical science and practice.

Mary and Joe should not forget this possibility or pass it by if it comes. But the greater danger is that the hope of improvement or even of complete restoration will occupy their lives to the exclusion of things more certain and will send them on a wasteful, wearying round among doctors good and bad. There will be plenty of quacks and charlatans to tempt them.

Given Joe's particular temperament, he will be especially susceptible to glowing promises of a cure. He will be wanting to try this, that, or something else, feverishly, impatiently, just because it will seem to be doing something. It will be up to Mary to curb this tendency, to keep him from squandering their time, energy, and slender means in pursuit of a probably illusory rainbow. She must see that neither of them sacrifices the quiet but solid worth of the present to a more exciting but wholly imagined future.

If he is physically hurt . . .
THE JOB'S THE THING

Betty and Dick

Not far from Mary on the station platform, leaning a thin shoulder against one of the pillars and staring thoughtfully down the tracks, stands Betty. She is waiting for Dick, to whom she has been engaged for three years, ever since he graduated from dental school and accepted a commission in the navy.

On his last furlough they made plans for getting married as soon as the war was over. "The next day after I get home?" Dick asked.

"Yes, or even the very day you come," Betty agreed.

Then one day only a few months ago came the word that Dick was wounded. A torpedo had struck the ship on which he worked as a dentist. Grateful that he had come through alive, Betty nevertheless was frantic with anxiety to hear from Dick himself. The letter, when it came, was written by someone else, a Red Cross social worker. "Don't worry about me," it began, "I'm okay—except for my good right arm, which got left somewhere in the Pacific."

Then a little farther on it read, "Guess maybe this means we'll have to reconsider those plans of ours. Maybe you'll want to change your mind. You'd have to count on dentist's bills now, you know. I'd understand if you just happened to have your heart set on a dentist for a husband."

The very casualness of it seemed almost more than Betty could bear. When Dick must be in despair. He worked so hard for his schooling, and his profession meant so much to him. Now that it was all lost, his hopes and plans in ruins, how could he think it would make any difference with her. Nobody could think that.

Yet when she told her father, he didn't seem so sure. "Well,

Betty," he said, "you know we think the world and all of Dick. We're proud of him, of course. But we must not be sentimental; we must face things squarely. You're only twenty-two, with your whole life ahead of you. I'm not sure I want to see you marry a . . ."

"Yes, father, a what?" Betty asked.

"Well, a . . . a one-armed man. There's no use beating around the bush, Betty. The fact is, Dick'll be a cripple!"

"I want to marry him more than ever now," Betty answered defiantly. "I'd want to marry him if he had lost two arms. He'll need me to take care of him now. And why not? I'm strong and healthy. I have a good job teaching school. Why shouldn't I work for us both, now that Dick can't?"

What's wrong with this picture?

As the preceding chapter may make you realize at once, there is a good deal wrong here. Betty's frame of mind, admirable in some ways, is a poor one in which to meet Dick and give him the kind of help he really needs. She and her father are about equally wrong in their reactions to the situation, because both of them are imagining a state of affairs that will not, or need not, exist. Dick will not be a cripple, and he is not going to be dependent on Betty to earn their living. Not, that is, unless he lets the loss of his arm spread in his mind until it seems that he has lost his legs too, not unless he lets himself become a cripple *in his mind*. And if he does show any tendency in this direction, Betty's natural and noble, but very mistaken, spirit of self-sacrifice won't help him reach a more healthy state of self-reliance.

She would do better, if necessary, to meet him with the story of the Minnesota banker who, though an accident deprived him of all his limbs except the stump of one hand, met life so successfully that he could and did say, with entire truth, "Thank God, I am not a cripple!" If this man—his name was Michael Dowling—could marry the belle of his town and provide her and their three daughters with something more than the comforts of life; if Charles McGonegal, who lost both his hands in World War I, can write, use the typewriter, shave himself, light his own cigarettes, drive his own car, fly his own airplane, and run his own ranch in California, then Betty's generosity and her father's fears are both unnecessary. All they need do is foster Dick's own determination to win through.

It is quite possible that Betty is in for a tremendous surprise when Dick arrives, for she is probably picturing him as thin and stooped, defeated-looking perhaps, and self-conscious about his empty sleeve, neatly folded and pinned inside his coat pocket. But the chances are at least even that Dick will step from the train as healthy and strong as ever, grinning happily as he looks around for Betty, having quite forgotten that he ever suggested she might want to change her mind.

For Dick has had several months in the care of the navy medical corps, and if he has been fortunate in the doctors he encountered and has been willing to cooperate with them, he may well have had an experience similar to that of Hilary Z.

One man's story

The piece of shell that struck Hilary in Italy did so much damage that the doctors had to amputate his left leg. The wound healed nicely and Hilary was soon as well physically as the doctors could make him. But they did not send him home, for he was gloomy and depressed, apathetic, indifferent. He had been a mail carrier in civilian days, and with a leg gone — well, what was there left?

Unless something was done about this attitude, the doctors knew, Hilary might sit out the rest of his life at home, a maimed hero, dependent on his pension and his family. To save his self-respect Hilary must be taught to work, and the sooner the better. So he was transferred to a convalescent hospital.

There the first step was to fit him with an artificial leg. Such a leg doesn't work of itself, and Hilary was inclined at first to think it more of a nuisance than anything else. He could manage better and much more comfortably on his crutches. But the doctors and nurses taught him how to use his upper thigh, hip, and back muscles to manipulate the leg, and, seeing the ease and efficiency with which some of the other fellows were getting around, even running and jumping, Hilary became more hopeful and more willing to co-operate in the program planned for him.

The counselors at the hospital studied his record, gave him several tests, and talked with him about his future. They described vocational possibilities that he had never dreamed of. His test record showed that he had a good deal of manual dexterity, so under their guidance he chose jewelry-making as his new occupation, and for several weeks he worked a scheduled number of hours each day at acquiring some of the elementary skills he would need for it. His progress was good, and gradually his interest mounted toward real enthusiasm.

Meanwhile, he was having fun. With the other fellows at the hospital—all of them wearing artificial limbs, braces, bandages, casts, or gadgets of one sort or another—he learned to dance again, to bowl, to play ping-pong, golf, handball, shuffleboard, and even tennis and baseball. His performance was hardly big-league style, of course, but it never had been, and he could still play well enough for pleasure and exercise.

With returning self-confidence in work and play, Hilary's gloom dropped away. He returned to something like his old self—whistling, wisecracking, griping, and arguing in about his normal proportions.

The staff then decided he was ready to begin his special training in earnest. So they arranged for him to enter a vocational training school near his home, where it would be possible for him to live with his family. He was discharged then, with the knowledge that when he had finished his course, the Veterans Administration or the USES would help him find a good job in a jewelry factory.

Hilary did not return home a discouraged, legless cripple, a burden to himself and to his family. He went home a whole man, once again hopeful, eager, optimistic. He had a handicap, yes. Some of his former activities were closed to him, and in others he tired more easily because even with proficiency it takes more effort to use an artificial leg than one's own. But there was nothing to prevent him from functioning again as a useful, self-reliant, happy man.

Because convalescent hospital facilities of this kind are limited, not all veterans who are rated partially disabled are as far along as Hilary in their rehabilitation before they return home. If they are not, their families, taking a cue from the way the doctors handled Hilary, can and should help them in their return from despair to hope.

Morale is half of it

Experience after experience, both civilian and military, has demonstrated the importance of this psychological factor in recovery. Industrial records show hundreds of accident cases in which the disability was severe and long out of all proportion to the extent of the physical damage, in spite of good treatment for the injured body. The difficulty was with morale; it was psychological, not physical.

Dr. Gordon Kamman tells a story of a British psychiatrist who in an argument with a surgeon friend during World War I wagered him a dinner that if he would carefully review the cases in his surgical wards he would find that 50 per cent of the suffering of his patients was caused by faulty psychological adjustment.

A few weeks later the surgeon took the psychiatrist to dinner. "When you said 50 per cent, you were putting it mildly," he admitted. "For instance, Corporal Smith had a kidney shot away by shrapnel. His wound was healed, his temperature and pulse were normal. But he wasn't doing well. He wasn't regaining his strength. He had no interest in life, no pep; couldn't eat. These weren't physical effects of the loss of a kidney. He was worrying about what would happen when he left the hospital. How would he get along with only one kidney? When we explained to him that his remaining kidney would enlarge to almost twice its normal size and take over the functions of the organ that was gone, so that he wouldn't even know he'd lost a kidney, he began to improve at once and now is up and around the wards.

"The same thing was true of Sergeant Clark, who had a leg shot off in action. The surgical wound was doing well, healing fine, but Clark wasn't getting along. He was weak, listless, had no appetite, wasn't gaining strength. There wasn't any physical reason for this; he was depressed by the social, economic, and cosmetic effects he thought would result from the loss of his leg. When we told him the government would give him a pension and an artificial leg and would find him a job when he got up and around, he began to get well and is now a different man."

This psychological factor is also present, though perhaps not so severe, in disabilities resulting from disease instead of injury. The man who has contracted tuberculosis, heart disease, malaria, stomach ulcer, or something similar has no visible disfigurement or deformity to complicate his social readjustment, but the restrictions his illness imposes upon him may well induce depression, bitterness, irritability, and lack of the will to try.

The incapacitating effects of most of these diseases are known to us because of their frequency among civilians. We know, for instance, that a man with tuberculosis, even when the disease has been arrested, must always conserve his strength to guard against a recurrence of the disease. We know that heart trouble in most of its forms is a bar to violent exertion, great excitement, undue tension.

Malaria, however, is less well known to Americans today, although it was a prevalent scourge in many areas during frontier days. In spite of the tremendously effective use of atabrine in combating this mosquito-borne infection, some veterans returning from the Pacific theater will have occasional bouts of it for a period of years.

The disabling effects of malaria lie in its tendency to recurrence. In roughly half the cases, it is not cured once and for all like pneumonia or a sore throat. It comes back again and again at varying intervals, because of changes of climate, temperature, or season, or for no apparent reason at all.

The periodic relapses are not dangerous if properly treated with quinine or atabrine, but they are highly unpleasant and they interfere with regular schedules of any kind. Each attack may last for several days, followed by a week or two of convalescence from the weakness left by the repeated succession of chills, fever, and profuse sweating. If the recurrences appear frequently, they may constitute a serious handicap in holding a job. It would be discouraging, to say the least, never to know whether, when you were planning a party, you would be able to go or would be in bed with an attack of malaria.

Fortunately, these recurrences do not continue throughout the victim's lifetime. Seldom do they trouble him for more than three or four years and in most cases not longer than a year or two.

Vocational retraining

In all cases of partial disability, whether from injury or disease, the heart of the individual's comeback will be his ability to secure and hold a suitable and satisfying job. The person with something useful and interesting to do will find his worries and nervous fears dwindling. "Work is nature's best medicine." And in this fundamental phase of rehabilitation, the kind of assistance and retraining given Hilary Z. is available to every disabled soldier with an honorable discharge if he needs it. To provide it is the chief function of the Veterans Administration.

Before a disabled man is discharged from any branch of the service he is given a special examination to determine as exactly as possible the nature and extent of his disability. The report of this examination together with his service record is sent to the rating board nearest his home at the time of his discharge. The rating board will determine the amount of pension to which he is entitled and also whether or not his disability constitutes a vocational handicap that makes him eligible for vocational retraining.

Every disabled veteran whose disability has been incurred in the line of military duty is entitled to a pension commensurate with his disability, but not every disabled man is eligible for retraining. It depends on whether or not he needs it—that is, whether or not his disability is the kind that would prevent his returning to his old kind of work.

For example, of two men each of whom has lost three fingers on his left hand, one might be rated eligible for retraining and the other not. The reason would be that the first man had been an insurance salesman, the second a violinist. The insurance salesman can do his work as well as before; the loss of his fingers is no vocational handicap for him, so he is not eligible for retraining in some other line of work. The violinist, however, could not go back to playing in an orchestra; the loss of his fingers *is* a vocational handicap, so he is eligible for retraining.

If a man is judged ineligible for retraining and for some reason thinks the decision is unjust, he may appeal to the rating board for a review of his case. If on either the first or this second consideration he is judged eligible, the board will send him an application blank to be filled out and sent in to the Veterans Administration.

What the receipt of this blank offers him is the chance to learn a new trade or profession at government expense. He may learn it in a business college, a trade school, or a university, or he may learn it "on the job," that is, by apprenticeship in some shop or factory or to some established workman such as a mechanic, a plumber, or a carpenter.

No veteran is compelled to take this retraining; it is only offered him. If he decides to accept the offer, he fills out the blank and sends it to the Veterans Administration office nearest his home.

In a few days he will receive a card or letter notifying him when to come to the office for an interview. There counselors will do for him what the hospital counselors did for Hilary Z.:

find out all they can about his special interests, abilities, and background training and experience. They may ask him to spend a day taking achievement, personality, and interests tests. Then on the basis of the information thus collected, they will discuss with him the job possibilities open to him and help him make a wise choice of the new occupation he is to learn. Once this decision has been reached—and it is the man himself who makes it; the counselors merely advise him—a good school or place of training is chosen, and his course begins.

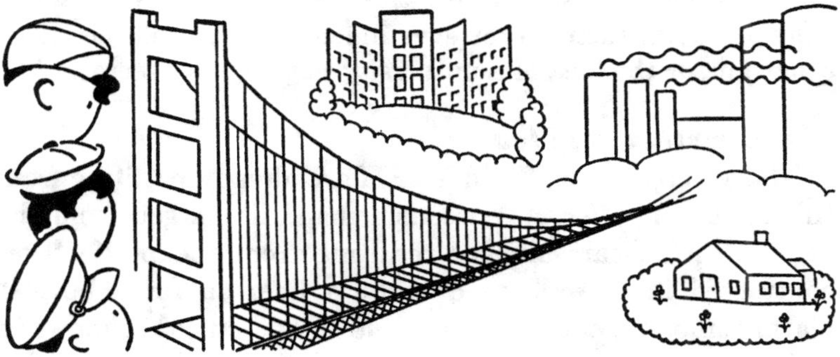

Vocational retraining: a bridge to the future

Of course, a man need not accept the counseling service of the Veterans Administration in order to get his retraining. If he knows exactly what he wants to do and what school he wishes to attend, the Veterans Administration will make the necessary arrangements for him. But he is entitled to the counselors' advice without charge; he has nothing to lose by hearing their suggestions.

Suppose he thinks he wants to go to the university and study journalism. How sure is he that he has the abilities needed for success in this field? It is just good sense to do what he can to find out before rather than after he has enrolled in the course. He need not be nervous or afraid about the tests he may be asked to take. They are not like the examinations he used to take in school; they don't determine his success or failure, nor do they in any way add to or subtract from his ability; they merely serve to make clearer the ability he has. If they should show that he has a high degree of mechanical dexterity but little facility in handling words, he would be well advised to go to a trade school rather than to the university.

Left to his own devices, the veteran is all too likely to pick some occupation, in radar or refrigeration perhaps, because he has heard rumors that it is a coming field and will pay good money. But it won't pay him good money if he can't do a good job in it. He will be happier and more successful if he finds out what his special abilities are and chooses a kind of work that fits them—however much more glamorous some other job, or the idea of a university degree, may seem.

It's more than an idea

Many veterans of World War II are already profiting from this retraining offer. A Wisconsin man, discharged from the army with a heart ailment resulting from rheumatic fever contracted in Hawaii, used to be a lineman for a burglar alarm company, climbing poles and in and out of windows to string or repair wires. His heart won't permit his doing this any longer, so he is following up an interest in electronic devices he got through his experience with the electric eye used in burglar alarms. He is studying electrical engineering at the state university.

Another man who came out of service with a bad heart used to work in a store for sixty dollars a month. Now he is drawing ninety-two dollars a month plus his part-time wages, while he learns on the job to be a shoemaker. Another was a truck driver before Pearl Harbor, but in the army he learned to repair radio and telegraph equipment, then to code and decode messages. He was discharged because of a severe glandular ailment called Hodgkin's disease. When he was well enough to fit himself for some sort of work, he wanted to take a university course in communications and his counselors agreed that he was fitted for it. But his doctors strongly advised against it as too great a strain on his weakened physical strength. So he is taking a shorter, less strenuous course in business college.

Then there's the case of a boy who had his appendix removed in an army hospital. A blood clot appeared in his leg after the operation, so he had to be discharged. He must still wear an elastic stocking on his leg and cannot go back to the welder's job he held before the war. He has a great deal of mechanical skill, so it was decided to apprentice him as a toolmaker in a factory in his home town. He can sit down at this job, and he is turning out to be a whiz at it.

These are only a few scattered examples of the new and often better start made possible by the vocational retraining program. Yet in spite of its manifest advantages, only a small proportion of those who are eligible for retraining are taking it.

There are many reasons for this. Some just don't care enough to make any extra effort. Others prefer to try their old job. Even though they have been rated eligible for retraining — which, as we have said, means that in the opinion of qualified judges their disability would be a handicap in their former job — they stubbornly cling to the kind of work they already know.

But probably the majority of those who do not take retraining, seeing that jobs are plentiful and wages good and having their pensions to help them out financially, prefer to get some job, any job, at once and not bother with special training. So they throw the application blank away. Or they may toss it aside not knowing what it is or means, thinking it's just "some more red tape." Later if jobs are harder to get or if when the rating board reviews their case, as it will once a year, it decides their condition is improved and cuts their pension, they may want retraining badly. But if the six-year limit set by law has passed, they will be too late to get it. They may not be so lucky as one man who discovered his error fairly soon. He went to the Veterans Administration office to see whether he could get a government loan to help him build a house.

"Are you getting any money from the government now?" asked the interviewer.

"Yes, twenty dollars a month." This told the interviewer that the man had a disability and might be entitled to retraining.

"Did you get any kind of blank to fill out?" he asked.

"Yes, I guess so. I don't know what it was, though. I'm so sick of red tape I didn't even read it."

The interviewer explained what the blank was and then asked the man about his job. He worked in a foundry, he said, the same place he worked before the war.

"Do you like the job? Do you want to go on working there?"

"No, I don't like it very well. It's harder for me, now that I've got this trouble. And my wife, she's crazy for me to get out of the foundry."

The interviewer set to work, soon the man was enrolled in a vocational school course in electrical repair work, and he and his wife were both much happier.

Wanted, a job

We may assume that those who go to the trouble of taking retraining are willing to work, want to work. Placing them in suitable jobs, if they have chosen their new occupation wisely and have finished their training successfully, will present little problem. The Veterans Administration placement officer of the USES will find jobs for them when their course is completed.

The USES placement services will be available also to those who do not elect to take training first. A number of USES interviewers have been regularly assigned to duty in the principal service hospitals to assist the disabled men who want to work immediately but who will be unable to return to their old civilian jobs. Their medical records are given careful consideration in finding suitable jobs for them.

Of course, these employment services can accomplish their task successfully only to the extent that our economic system functions properly to make sufficient jobs available. Some of our leaders are on the right track in emphasizing the importance of providing enough productive jobs to go around, for returning servicemen as well as for those who have served on the home front.

We owe the handicapped, even more than the unimpaired, a debt we can never satisfactorily repay, but we can come closest to repayment by getting them back into the ordinary stream of civilian life as quickly as possible. Adequate pensions are justified as props to their morale until they can re-establish themselves, but for the man's own sake the pension should not be so large or so long continued as to be a cushion on which he can rest through life.

Money is the easier gift, but a way to sound mental health is more important and more valuable. "A place to sleep, enough food for the belly, and enough clothing to keep out the cold has never yet been enough to save a man's soul." Those who have lived long with a crippling disability know whereof they speak when they say to the newly handicapped, as they invariably do when asked for advice, "Get ready to work. If work is at all possible, you won't be happy without it."

Of course, among the handicapped as among the unimpaired, there will be some who won't want to work, who will feel that they have earned the right to a living at society's expense. Veterans of this sort were much in the news after World War I. New York City newspapers, for instance, were greatly concerned about the number of young men still in uniform who were peddling apples, shoestrings, or "welcome home" banners from house to house or at busy downtown intersections.

Knowing that the country's economic machinery was creaking badly and that jobs were by no means plentiful, the editors assumed that these young men had resorted to what was really begging because they could find no work. So with indignant sympathy they pointed out the irony of the situation: New York City had staged for its returning soldiers a gigantic welcoming spectacle that cost several thousands of dollars, then a few weeks later it generously instructed its policemen not to arrest wounded soldiers for peddling shoestrings without a license!

Investigation, however, showed that comparatively few of the peddlers knew no other way of earning a living, and for these men jobs were soon found. The others did not want jobs; they had discovered they could get more and easier money by peddling. One of them boldly admitted to the investigator, "Why should I work? I made fifty dollars yesterday selling 'welcome home' buttons." These men had learned that their uniforms and their crutches and bandages — though by no means all of them were disabled — would win them easy money from the many whose pity is quick but untempered by insight or wisdom.

Self-respecting servicemen were not at all pleased by this superficial and symbolic appreciation on the part of the public. The *American Legion Weekly* warned the people against these "Peddlers in Uniform": Do not buy from them in the belief that you are showing appreciation for all men who were in service. Instead you are helping to support an abuse that is resented by servicemen generally. But the warning had little effect. The general public, in a hurry and much preoccupied with its own affairs, finds it much easier to satisfy its sense of obligation by tossing a dime or a dollar to an individual than to do something constructive about the slower and more complex process of sound rehabilitation.

Colonel William C. Menninger, one of the division chiefs in the office of the surgeon general during World War II, has issued some advice to the public: "Civilians should put their relations with veterans on a realistic basis. They should recognize that the servicemen have risked a great deal but that doesn't make them gods. Put it this way: The civilian owes a debt to the soldier, but that doesn't mean the civilian should be indulgent and regard the soldier like a spoiled child."

This attitude is as applicable to the handicapped as to the nonhandicapped. Most of them will not act like spoiled children and will resent being treated as if they were. The others, those who expect an easy living, who cheerfully or whiningly let themselves be supported by others without effort on their part, who noisily and vehemently insist on all sorts of special privileges and dispensations because they are disabled veterans, who work much harder to prove themselves eligible for large pensions than to make themselves independent of any pension — these men will challenge the wisdom, intelligence, and tact, individually of their own family and friends, collectively of society as a whole. Their will to work, their desire for self-respecting independence, must be established as quickly as possible. In dealing with these men especially, sentimentality is barred. Give their self-pity so much as a teardrop to feed on and it will flourish like a weed.

The time element is important. The habit of dependence, of riding on another's back, is quickly formed, and once set it is not easily broken. A couple of years ago a man in Connecticut tried an experiment with some veterans of World War I who were living in a veterans' home. He wanted to see what could be done to help them back to self-support. Selecting those who were physically capable of working, he enrolled them in training courses of one sort or another, and supplied them with whatever was necessary in the way of working clothes, tools, and transportation.

Three quarters of the group completed the course successfully, and of these 90 per cent were offered suitable jobs at an average wage of forty-two dollars a week. Yet the experiment was almost a complete failure. Some of the men did not even investigate the job offered to them. Others failed to report for work after they were hired. Still others accepted work but quit after a couple of weeks or a month or two. Only 30 per cent were faithful workers for three months or more. The rest had been idle dependents on charity for too long. It is significant that for most of them the training was not the stumbling block; their ability to learn was still present. It was their will to work, their will to support themselves, that was gone.

Look at the record

The other side of this job question is, of course, the willingness of business and industry to employ the handicapped. And on this score, the evidence indicates, the veteran need have little fear. The working world is by no means unacquainted with the disabled employee; it met him during and after World War I, got to know him better through state and federal agencies for the rehabilitation of the civilian handicapped, and has welcomed him in increasing numbers during the manpower shortage of World War II.

Much of this experience has been rather hit-or-miss, without over-all plan or careful analysis, yet it has taught employers that handicapped persons can be useful and efficient workers, that not every job requires the use of all a man's limbs or all his senses.

They have learned, for instance, that a man with an artificial leg can run a rivet squeezer (or any one of a hundred other machines) perfectly well; all he needs is a stool on which to rest his artificial leg while the other foot presses the pedal. They have learned that neither speech nor hearing is needed for assembling radio parts, or for sorting and distributing materials. They have learned that the disabled are often, indeed, at an advantage in some operations or departments — as, for instance, the deafened in departments where boilermaking is carried on or where saws cut shriekingly through sheet metal.

"Won't our accident rate go up if we hire handicapped workers?" used to be the question most often asked. Not any more, for the record shows that the accident rate goes down, that the handicapped have fewer accidents because, as one employer put it, "They're not so damned reckless."

Testimony to this effect by employers in many different branches of industry is presented in two recent pamphlets, one issued by the National Office of Education, the other by the Civil Service Commission. These same employers declare that the records of the handicapped in absenteeism, tardiness, and turnover are strikingly better than those of the able-bodied; that they are conscientious, superior workers; that they expect no favors, and produce as well or better than the average of the nonhandicapped. Perhaps this is true because their jobs mean more to them, or perhaps because in overcoming the social and psychological effects of their disability they have learned a greater measure of self-discipline.

This experience has pointed the way for the intelligent placement of disabled veterans in jobs where they can be useful and productive. Industrial leaders as well as government agencies have foreseen the problem and are devising procedures for meeting it. Many of the bigger industrial units, by a careful analysis of every operation performed in their various plants, know the exact physical requirements of each and every job they have to fill. Westinghouse Electric, for instance, knows that in its manufacturing divisions 83 per cent of the jobs can be done by one-eyed men, 82 per cent by deaf men, 19 per cent by one-legged men, 17 per cent by men who use canes or crutches, and so on.

Such an analysis is, of course, only the first step in the process. Once it has been completed and its results are tabulated or conveniently coded, special procedures are set up to make sure that, in so far as possible, the right man and the right job are brought together. The final aim is to match the physical capacities of a given individual with the physical requirements of a given job.

Fitting the man with the job

It is true that this planned, systematic approach to the efficient employment of the handicapped is still pretty much confined to the larger industrial plants. But their managers are taking the lead, through conferences and round table discussions of many sorts, in spreading the results of their experience through the ranks of business and industry, so that similar methods may prevail in smaller plants and among less farsighted and aggressive employers.

Nor is it only their methods they are seeking to pass along. They are also, perhaps primarily, interested in instilling sound attitudes toward this whole matter. Much of their emphasis is on correcting the attitude of the employer who says, or thinks, "Poor Jack. It's too bad he lost an arm in the war. What say we give him a job as a watchman? That'll help him out. We've got to be good to the boys who fought for us, you know."

This man's heart may be in the right place, but his mind is not. The hiring of a disabled veteran should not be, and in most cases is not, a matter of dispensing charity. It is a matter to be dealt with factually, not sentimentally, in a straightforward businesslike manner, not in a mist of mistaken altruism.

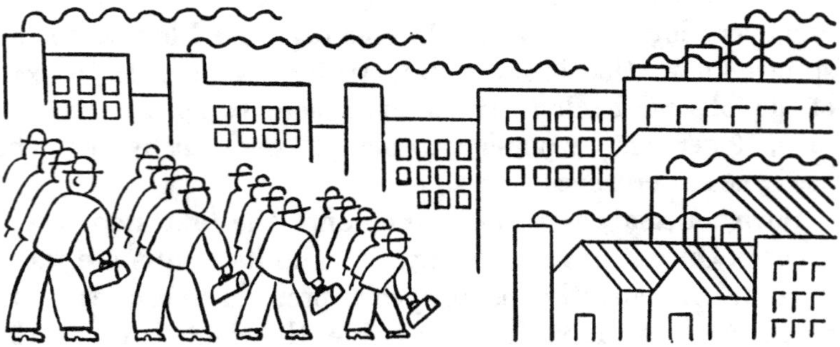

A job is his right!

In the first place, Jack deserves and is definitely capable of something better than going on guard, sweeping floors, and the like. Most of his original ability as a worker still remains, and he should be employed where this remaining skill can best be used. Any other solution is a social waste of manpower that should not be tolerated.

In the second place, if a man is so disabled that he must be pensioned, it is not industry's task to provide the pension. That is society's responsibility. The cost should be borne by the taxpayers as a whole, not by a limited number of consumers who must pay in higher prices the cost of inefficiency in the production of the goods they buy.

The employing of handicapped workers is not a great problem; it is rather a question of correct procedures. The disabled man who seeks work is not disabled in all his functions, only in part of them. Therefore, properly placed in a job that he can do in a normal and satisfactory manner, *he is not handicapped on that job,* however severely disabled he may be otherwise.

The problem then, for any employer, is one of correct placement, of fitting the man with the job — a procedure that should be customary in the employment of anybody, whether handicapped or not. A wise employer does not make a foreman out of a man who can't get along with people, or a janitor out of a born salesman, or a file clerk out of a girl who must stop to think whether *d* comes before or after *e*. Neither will the wise employer put an arrested case of tuberculosis on a job as a battery repairman, where he would be exposed to the fumes of various gases; or in a packing plant, exposed to sudden changes of temperature going in and out of refrigerators; or in a flour mill or a mine, exposed to flour and coal dust. Nor will he place a man with an injured back on a job that requires heavy lifting.

In *all* cases the wise employer's policy will be to match the requirements of the job with the determinable abilities and disabilities of the individual. Instead of disqualifying the handicapped man because of his disability, the employer will learn how best to qualify him because of his abilities.

Such accurate and selective placement usually involves consideration of more than purely physical factors. Indeed, some industrial leaders believe that proper regard for nervous and emotional factors, called "environmental placement," is the most important single consideration in the proper placement of returning soldiers, whether they are physically disabled or not. They would not ask a man wounded by a gun shot to work in an armament crib, or a veteran who spent three years in an enemy prison camp to work long hours in a small space tightly enclosed by massive machinery.

Good environmental placement may tax the ingenuity and the patience of the employment staff. One man back from combat, his physical injuries healed, was put first in a department where riveting was being done. The noise was too much like the machine guns; he couldn't take it. He was transferred to the office, but here the driving noise of the typewriters got him. So he was transferred back to the factory, but this time to a quiet place inspecting materials. Here his jitters left him and his work record was very good.

Such men are not just being fussy and unreasonable. They cannot help their frayed nerves, and employers can help a great deal by a little extra effort in placing them.

Don't judge by the misfits

Among the disabled veterans as well as among the others there will be some misfits, men for whom no amount of effort seemingly will find a satisfactory job. Probably investigation would show that their service record was bad, and their pre-war record too.

Industry cannot be expected to bear the burden of their maladjustment, and in most cases it won't have to; these are the men who quit voluntarily and wander on, aimlessly, restlessly. But it certainly is not fair for an employer to react as one did after an encounter with a disabled veteran of this type. Angrily he phoned the employment service. "Don't send me any more of these wounded men. They're no good." His childishness is obvious. After all, is there not the same percentage of misfits among civilians as among veterans?

The correct attitude is the same for employers as for anyone else: Treat the disabled veterans as human beings. Forget they are veterans. Give them the same chance you would any other man. Get away from the notion that they are any different from the rest of the community.

Failing to take this attitude, some manufacturers have been fearful about hiring the returned soldier whose discharge is labeled "medical." They can see nothing the matter with him but they feel there must be something wrong, so they start trying to find out what it is. This is a mistaken approach. They should give the veteran who comes for a job exactly the same physical examination as they would to any other person, and if nothing shows up they should hire him on the same terms as they would a civilian. Many medical discharges are for minor physical difficulties that would be a disability for army service but not for employment in industry. Flat feet, for instance. Or, as in one case, an allergy to wool.

The military authorities have persistently refused to make available to employers or employment agencies the diagnosis that lies behind the medical discharge. They feel that the physical standards of the armed services are so much more severe than those in industry that if the results of army or navy examinations were made known, the veteran would be penalized in competition with civilian applicants for jobs. For the veteran's own sake, however, so that he may not be placed in a job that will do him harm, the army and navy medical corps do inform employment services of the limitations, if any, which the man's disability may impose on the type of work he should do. Beyond this neither more nor less of physical and mental wholeness should be required of veterans than of civilians.

No concessions asked

The employer cannot alone achieve success in this policy of correct placement; the employee must be willing to cooperate. He must be willing to accept the limitations imposed by his handicap, take the job he can do, and not yearn for one that is beyond his reach at the moment.

In some plants where the kind of placement service we have described has been tried, the handicapped themselves have sometimes nullified its benefits by ingenious ways of circumventing the arrangements made for them. They have managed slyly to get themselves transferred to another job without consulting the placement personnel. In some cases the new job proved hazardous for them and the results were disastrous.

If the man has good and sufficient reason for wanting to

be transferred he will probably find the placement staff quite willing to arrange it, so long as the new job is within his capacities. And it is as much to his advantage as to his employer's that he do work in which his disability is not a handicap.

If the employer is not to consider his hiring of the handicapped an act of charity, neither must the employee. That is, he must accept his responsibility for full and efficient production in whatever job he is hired for. He must not accept his wages as a pension, trade on his handicap, and try to get by with as little effort as possible. He must not expect his foreman or his office supervisor to make allowances for his handicap. The proper place for such allowances is in the selection of the job, not on the job itself. If allowances are necessary, the job is not the right one and the man himself, if he is forthright and honest, will request a transfer. He will not consider or ask others to consider his disability an excuse for poor or inefficient work.

Dr. Earl Carlson was a victim of spastic paralysis (an affliction in which the muscles of the arms or the legs or both are held tight in a state of tension, so that under excitement or stimulation they shake or tremble). He had with great determination and effort overcome the disability sufficiently to attend medical school. One of his professors was strict about requiring precise and complete knowledge and in consequence was greatly feared by his students. When called on to recite one day, Carlson was embarrassed at not knowing the full answer to the question and his spasticity reasserted itself. Twitching and shaking miserably, he sat down.

The professor immediately commanded him to stand up. "Don't think for a minute, Carlson," he said, "that just because you are a cripple you can afford to be sloppy in your studies. I refuse to make any exceptions for you."

This, of course, sounds cruel, but in the long run it was kind. Carlson was trying to make his own way in life, and if he was to succeed he must be able to meet other doctors as an equal. The world of science and medicine can make no exceptions for physical disability, and the professor's seeming cruelty helped Dr. Carlson to meet that world on its own terms, making no allowances for himself and asking from others no special considerations or privileges.

As this story suggests, the disabled man's chief task, if he is to achieve success in the working world, is to win the battle with himself. Employers testify that the major difficulty with the handicapped as employees is in their personal relationships. They imagine all sorts of things. If they are deaf they think the other employees are whispering about them. If they stutter, they think the others make fun of them. If they are disfigured, they are sure their fellow workers shun them or slight them. They build ordinary thoughtlessness into deliberate insults. Or they are self-conscious and appear self-pitying.

A man who had lost a hand in the war went to ask for a job with his sleeve pinned into the pocket of his coat. One could tell from the newness of his suit that he had just been discharged.

The employer, who had been without one hand for twenty-five years, looked at the man standing defeated and miserable before him and said, "Well, did they get you in the head too? The way you've got your sleeve pinned in there and the way you act, it looks like they did. Sure, I've got a job for you, but not if you're going to go around feeling sorry for yourself. Not unless you want to work instead of just sitting around having someone wait on you. Go back and have them fit you with a new hand. And if you don't like it, do what I did: learn to use the other one."

It is in this battle with himself that the family and friends can help the veteran. In most cases they cannot do much about getting him a job or fitting him into the right one; that is up to him and his employer. But they can help him overcome his depression and his fears. They can give him moral support while he struggles against discouragement to learn his new work. They can help him to feel wanted and useful, to forget himself and his disability in new interests, in fun and recreation, in warm companionship with others.

Some do's and don'ts

The principles given for the guidance of family and friends on pages 57 to 67 are as applicable to the partially disabled as to those more severely handicapped. The differences between these two groups are of degree rather than of kind.

The problem will, of course, vary with the individual. Among both the completely and the partially disabled there will be some whose will to do must be strengthened and some in whom it must be toned down. In general, however, those as severely injured as Joe, especially if they have his active, impatient temperament, will need help in curbing their ambitions, in accepting the limitations of their disability, in channeling their energies into quieter occupations and pleasures. Whereas a man with an arm missing, like Dick, or otherwise partially handicapped will be more likely to need showing that his life has not narrowed as much as he thinks it has, that his life is not over, that he has much more left than he has lost.

Slumps in morale will unaccountably hit some of these men harder than others. They will feel despair out of all proportion to the extent of their injury. One case has been reported in which a man who had lost an arm planned to commit suicide. He didn't want his wife to have to take care of him, and he could not imagine being able to take care of himself any longer. His whole life, all his abilities, seemed tied up in the use of the arm he had lost. He could think of nothing left to him that he could enjoy. So he planned to take his own life as soon as he could get out of the hospital and be sure that his attempt would succeed.

Fortunately, those who were taking care of him sensed the depth of his despair and did something about it. They arranged that he should see and talk with men worse off than he who were having a good time in spite of their handicaps, that he should hear and read about handicapped men who have achieved signal success in art, in science, in business. Gradually he came to see how absurd his attitude was. "I got some sense," he said. "I began to try." And he found before long that he was doing almost all the things he had previously done with both his arms.

Don't let his handicap spread above his shoulders. Don't let the physical disability become a mental handicap. Take full account, that is, of the psychological factors involved in his recovery. Never underestimate their importance.

Dick and those like him will have to face the same difficult transition from soldier to civilian as Tom in our first story, plus the additional problems resulting from their handicaps. They will have the same cause for restlessness and bitterness, plus the concrete evidence to remind them of it. They will feel the same lack of preparedness for a satisfying job, with less equipment with which to prepare. They will have the same desperate need to fit quietly back into the stream of civilian life, but they will be less able to do so because they will feel more conspicuous and different.

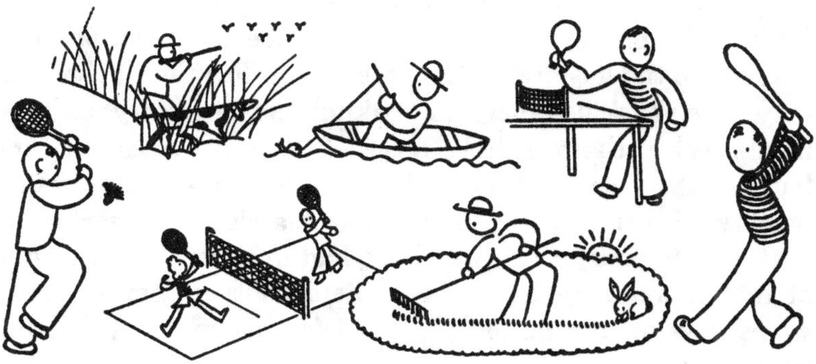

Good medicine for low morale

In helping them through this difficult adjustment, keep in mind the value of games, exercise, entertainment, and social good times. Especially if they show an inclination to remain on the sick list too long, diversion of any kind from their brooding and jolly, amiable companionship will be of incalculable assistance. Learning again to participate in athletic games—tennis, baseball, handball, archery, bait and fly casting, darts, badminton, horseshoes, swimming, tumbling, and wrestling will all be possible for most of them—

will not only give their morale the much-needed boost but, if properly selected according to their handicap, will strengthen and train the muscles made weak and flabby by disuse.

It goes without saying that the wife or mother is not going to help the veteran keep his eye upon the doughnut if she herself sees only the hole. If she thinks his life is over, that he must be an invalid waited upon hand and foot the rest of his days, she will only aggravate his problem. He will have to fight her then as well as himself, and the odds will be great against his winning through to independence.

In one area a special word of encouragement can be given. The veteran, and his wife too, may think that because he has lost one or more of his limbs, they can no longer have satisfactory sexual relations. Amputation may make it necessary for them to learn new techniques and methods for intercourse, but these adjustments are not too difficult.

Special attention is given to this important matter in military hospitals, and in many cases the wives are invited to come to the hospital so that they as well as their husbands may receive skilled help in making the necessary adjustments. When the men have returned from convalescent furloughs, they are encouraged to discuss their experience frankly with the doctor and the psychiatric social worker so that any difficulty they may have had in their first attempts at intercourse may be corrected before either they or their wives develop the notion that satisfaction in the act is no longer possible.

However, if this problem has not been solved before the man is discharged, the wife should seek advice and instruction from a psychiatrist or from a psychiatric social worker on the staff of the Red Cross or the family welfare agency. The continued success of her marriage may depend on her being able to face the sexual situation with confidence, secure in the knowledge that her husband's disability need not disturb this phase of their relationship.

Make full use of the facilities set up to help him. The Veterans Administration, the United States Employment Service, the Red Cross, the various service organizations — these and a host of other agencies offer to you and to him advice and suggestions born of experience and special training in the situations you must meet. Do not hesitate to seek their help when you need it, whether the immediate problem is a major psychological crisis or some smaller question such as where to turn for a special service of some kind, a special appliance, or the like.

When you go to such agencies for information or advice, remember that the aim of all of them and of their staff members is to help the veteran achieve the greatest possible measure of mental, social, and economic self-sufficiency. They will work with all their knowledge and resources to this end. If this is not what you want, do not go. You will merely waste their time and rob someone else of their services. But don't then say there is no help for you. The truth is that you don't really want help; you want money or some other means of transferring your load to other shoulders.

Don't spend too much time and effort on his pension claims. In most cases there should be no trouble about the disabled veteran's pension. The process of award will be almost automatic, and the rating board's decision will be satisfactory. But in any decision that rests somewhat upon judgment and not entirely on rule, there is room for honest differences of opinion. If you are convinced that there has been some error or misunderstanding of the circumstances in your soldier's case, he is entitled to ask for a reconsideration and should do so.

But do not let him — and especially do not *urge* him — to go beyond this legitimate effort to secure what he believes he is entitled to. One man who was getting sixty dollars a month for a partial disability was so bothered by the notion that he deserved more that it interferred with his work. He was getting on nicely with his job, but he kept asking the company doctor to give him a letter to the rating board saying he should have more pension. When the doctor firmly refused, pointing to his good attendance and production record in the plant, the man began to be absent more and more frequently, claiming he was too ill to work.

Others have gone to even greater lengths, spending a great deal of time, energy, and ingenuity in devising schemes for proving their eligibility for bigger monthly checks from the government. If they had expended half as much effort on a job, they would not have needed any pension. At the end of such a road lies mental and moral sickness.

On the other hand, some disabled men have refused to accept the pensions granted them. They seem to consider the payments a kind of dole, which they are too proud to accept. If this attitude does not result from a refusal to accept the fact of their disability, it is perhaps better for their mental health and strength than the other extreme, but it is still quixotic. The middle road is the one of common sense: Accept what is due you, consider it a resource against a rainy day, and then work to free yourself from either financial or psychological dependence on it.

If for some reason it becomes necessary for your man to file a claim for a pension, *do not let an outsider do it for him*. Shysters of all sorts sprang up after World War I, and will probably do so again, to grow fat at the expense of disabled veterans. They will promise to get Tom, Dick, or Harry a pension because they "know the ropes," or because they "have influence," or on some other pretext. Then they will claim a good fat fee or a percentage of the pension checks.

If your husband or son or brother is not entitled to a pension, no such person can get it for him; and if he is eligible for one, he does not need any such "agent" to get it for him. These men have no special influence, rather the reverse, and there are no particular ropes to know. All that is needed is a statement of his case to someone at the Veterans Administration or to a representative of one of the service organizations or the Red Cross, and this person, *without charge*, will file the claim if there is any justification for it.

Don't let him, or in any way encourage him, to become a "professional veteran." A "professional veteran," as the term suggests, is one who makes a profession of being a veteran, who spends much or most of his time and energy in getting everything he can out of being a veteran. He not only will go to absurd lengths to demonstrate his eligibility for a pension, but he will claim special privileges and dispensations at every turn—from his family, his employer, his fellow workers, and society in general—just because he is a veteran. He will never let anyone forget what he did for his country, the sacrifices he made, the hardships he endured, the heroism he displayed.

The chances are, of course, that the records of such men would not bear much investigation. The men who really sacrificed, endured, and were heroic are the least likely to make capital of the fact. And these men, the real heroes, are the first to recognize and to scorn the professional veteran. They know that he is the worst enemy of the true interest of all veterans; he is likely to stigmatize the whole group.

It does not by any means require a disability of any sort to make a professional veteran. But the disabled man may be peculiarly tempted to this role because he has such a good peg on which to hang his claims. He has a handicap to dramatize and exploit. So do all you can to de-veteranize your disabled serviceman as quickly as possible, to get him thinking and feeling himself a civilian again. Help him to feel that, whatever his country may owe him, all he wants of it is what it owes to every citizen: the chance to help himself.

Remember that rewarding, productive work will be his best medicine. Urge him to find a job, not just any job, but one in which his disability will not be a handicap and in which he will feel useful and capable. On the job, of course, you must leave him to his employer and his fellow workers, but at home you can give him the comfort, encouragement, and moral support he will need while he struggles to find his niche and fit himself into it.

Finding the right job is tremendously important, and the first one may not be the right one. It must be given a fair trial, and the man must be sure the difficulty is with the job and not with himself before he leaves it, but if it does not get easier and he is not happier in it as time passes, then do not let him hesitate to change.

Making use of the various advisory services available should prevent his having to make a trial-and-error hunt, but if he insists on finding his own job without such advice, don't let him give up in despair if the first work he tries proves too much for him.

One discharged marine had a shoulder so badly injured on Guadalcanal that he could no longer lift, stretch, push, or reach. His first job was lifting airplane propellers; he could not do it, and he lost the job. He got another pulling a heavy cart around in a factory. This was no good either, and he was fired again. After losing two more jobs because they were not suited to his capacities now, he got very discouraged, thinking he would never find work he could do. But he tried once more, this time sitting at a table assembling camera parts with his fingers, and now he is happy and contented again.

If he is mentally hurt . . .

HE TOO IS ILL

Sarah and Ted

Older by some years than the others on the platform, Sarah, the fourth of the waiting women, keeps herself apart from them. She is a small woman, plain but meticulously neat in appearance. The worry and anxiety to be read in her face are apparent also in her nervous pacing across the far end of the platform, in the tense way she clutches her purse and knots and unknots her handkerchief. She is waiting for her son Ted, twenty-six years old, coming home from the army hospital in which he has been under treatment for some three months.

It was two weeks ago that the news came, the news that seemed to turn the world upside down for Sarah. Ever since, her heart has been torn by conflicting emotions, her brain racked with frantic thoughts. Ted was to be discharged, his army doctors said, but they felt he must have further treatment. Since the Veterans Administration hospital had no beds available, they were requesting her permission and co-operation in transferring him to the state hospital near his home.

It was the name of the hospital they wanted to send him to that turned Sarah's very blood to ice. That split second of realization seems burned upon her memory. Everything around her stood out in sharp outline: the faded pattern in the carpet, the half-empty coffee cup on the table beside her, dust in the shaft of sunlight from the window showing like hoarfrost on the green plush of the overstuffed chair.

They wanted to send Ted to the state hospital for the insane, which she and everyone else for miles around calls the asylum, or the madhouse, or the "bughouse."

Sarah thought Ted was in the hospital because he was ill;

but if this is where the doctors want to send him, they must think he is insane. It can't be so. Not Ted. Not the quiet, gentle, loving, and lovable boy who was her eldest and her favorite child, whom everybody liked because he was so agreeable, so kind, so good. He was always so helpful and obedient; he never got into trouble at school as her other children did.

Ted had the best mind too. She never could make Mary or Ruth or Jack settle down to their books and study. They always wanted to be out tearing around like wild Indians, getting into all kinds of mischief, playing hooky from school. But Ted loved to read for hours at a time, or to ramble through the woods hunting flower specimens for his collection or trying to find some new kind of bird. He had done very well in his studies, and as a high school teacher too, after he graduated from the teachers' college.

It was true that his principals sometimes complained about the way Ted taught; they didn't think he was strict enough in his discipline. But the boys and girls loved him, and he could make them learn.

What *could* have happened to Ted's mind?

Turning her back to the others on the platform to look out across the tops of the city buildings, Sarah, for the hundredth time, thinks over the events of Ted's furlough six months ago. There was nothing wrong with him then, nothing that didn't seem natural to Sarah when she remembered that he was tired and that he probably enjoyed being alone with the family after a year in the army. He hadn't wanted to meet people. Even the time he went downtown especially to get a haircut, he wouldn't go into the barbershop when he got there; he didn't want to talk to the barber, he said. And he wouldn't go into the butcher shop either, even to help Ruth carry the turkey, heavy as it was.

How they'd all laughed at his sudden dislike for yellow. Anything yellow made him angry, even the little ribbon Ruth wore in her hair. And once when they had rutabagas for dinner, he left the table, wouldn't eat.

He didn't talk much about his experiences in the army, but Sarah knew he didn't like the life. Some of the things he had to do bothered him. Once he had told her about his job of guarding prisoners. If they didn't do what he told them to, he was supposed to shoot at their legs. But he couldn't do it. "I just couldn't, Mom," he said. "They were just boys, like the kids I had in high school." But then he was punished for not obeying orders.

When Ted went into the army, Sarah was afraid he wouldn't make a good fighter, he was so tenderhearted. But during his furlough he said he wanted to get overseas. He wouldn't mind meeting the enemy with a bayonet face to face, he remarked over and over again, just so they didn't come up behind him. "You've got to get the enemy before they get you."

Certainly, Sarah thinks for the hundredth time, there was nothing insane or crazy about Ted then. Something terrible must have happened after he went back to camp.

Straightening her shoulders and facing about toward the others again, Sarah is sure once more that she has made the right decision. Whatever has happened, they aren't going to put Ted away in an asylum. She can spare him, and herself, that disgrace. She will take care of him at home. In spite of all the attempts to persuade her, she has refused to have Ted sent to the state hospital and insisted that the army authorities send him home to her instead.

So Sarah waits for Ted, her mind busy, as it has been so often these past two weeks, with ways and means of concealing the truth from her friends and neighbors—if Ted is what the doctors think he is. But somehow she is sure the doctors are wrong, that Ted's trouble will disappear with a few weeks of rest at home with her. "It will all blow over," she says to herself. "It must!"

Fear of the unfamiliar

Sarah's anguished distress is very real, but much of it is quite unnecessary. She is not so troubled because *something* has happened to Ted, but because of *what* has happened to Ted. She would feel and act very differently if he were being discharged because of a shrapnel wound or because he had contracted tuberculosis or had some heart disease. She would be sorry and disturbed of course, but she would not feel horrified and disgraced and be searching for ways of keeping the truth from the neighbors. She would not be questioning the doctors' diagnosis and refusing to help them give Ted the further care and treatment he needs. She is doing these things because Ted's illness or injury is of the mind.

Sarah would accept a disordered stomach or heart as entirely respectable, but she, in company with thousands of other uninformed people, considers a disordered mind something to be ashamed of, to be concealed at all costs.

This attitude is a hundred years out of date. It is based on ignorance, on lack of information or misinformation about mental illness, about the methods and institutions available for treating it, even about the medical specialists called psychiatrists who are trained to deal with it. And this ignorance can lead to disaster, as it did with George.

George's father died when he was ten, his mother when he was fifteen. They didn't leave much money behind, but George managed to work his way through the rest of high school and through college, graduating from one of our leading state universities with an honors degree in chemistry. He got a good job in the research department of a large drug company, and by his intelligence and hard work earned several promotions in quick succession.

Then the strain of his lonely life, of too much work and too little play, began to tell on him. He grew tense and jittery, couldn't sleep, suffered from increasingly severe headaches, and seemed unable to concentrate on his work as well as he had. Not understanding the cause of all this, he began to worry. Could he be losing his mind?

George had never been one to talk to others about himself or his problems, and he had not allowed himself much time for friendship. But he had an exceedingly likable personality, so that his teachers and now his employers took more than usual interest in him and his welfare. One day his boss, a sophisticated man of the world, talked to him about the fact that he seemed to have no women in his life. He ought to do something about this, said his boss; it wasn't normal.

The boss did not know, and George did not remember, the real answer to this: that so far it had taken all his time and money to get an education and get settled in a job. Instead, already feeling that he must be different from other people, George seized upon the idea that he wasn't normal. His fears and worries multiplied, his sleep grew more disturbed, his headaches worse.

The headaches finally sent him to a doctor. The doctor could find no physical injury or disease and suspected that George's symptoms were psychological in origin—that is, that the disorder in his mind was upsetting the physiology of his body. His organs were whole and undiseased, but the turmoil in his mind was preventing them from functioning properly.

Unfortunately, the doctor did not explain this to George. He simply recommended that he see a psychiatrist.

George had no real knowledge of what a psychiatrist is or does. He had only the idea that psychiatrists deal with insanity. So the doctor's recommendation simply convinced him that what he had feared was true; he was going insane.

In that case he knew what to do. He would not see a psychiatrist. Nor would he wait until he had lost his mind. Two weeks later he took his own life.

Ignorance isn't bliss

The real cause of George's death was ignorance. All his education had not given him the most elementary knowledge of how the mind works, of the many and varied illnesses to which it is subject, or of the treatment available for them. His knowledge and experience included only one kind of mental illness: what he had learned to call insanity. If he had been suffering from indigestion he would not have concluded immediately that he had cancer of the stomach, but at the first suggestion that something was out of order in his mind, he jumped to the conclusion that he was going insane. And once he had reached this conclusion, the stigma attached to mental disease came into play, along with the mistaken notion that insanity is incurable, to make his trouble seem a disaster and disgrace too great to be borne.

These same false notions are the principal source of Sarah's frantic anxiety about Ted.

The social stigma that plays so large a part in this process is a survival of the attitude that prevailed a century and more ago, before it was known that insanity is an illness. At that time people who had seriously disordered minds were thought to be possessed by devils or demons. They were not considered human beings or treated as such. They were objects sometimes of fun, sometimes of fear. So they were chained in dungeons or in cellars or haylofts, ridiculed and exhibited as monsters, tormented, tortured, flogged.

Advance in scientific knowledge has long since done away with these superstitious notions and with such cruelly inhuman treatment. Psychologists and physicians have come to understand what is wrong with these people, have come to know that they are suffering from an illness which may occur in many different forms and degrees of severity and which can often be cured. With this understanding have come greatly improved methods of treatment. Many cases of mental illness do not require institutional care at all, and for those that do, the old insane or lunatic asylum has been replaced by real hospitals for the mentally ill, hospitals staffed with doctors and nurses who have special training in diseases of the mind.

Thus on the level of science and medical practice mental illness has taken its proper place alongside physical illness. But the attitudes and understanding of the lay public have lagged far behind. We no longer believe in possession by demons, but we sometimes feel and act as though we did. We still lump all the mentally ill together as insane and picture them as raving, dishevelled creatures who don't know who they are or where. We still think of mental hospitals in terms of barred windows, strait jackets, shadowy corridors, and wild laughter.

Nothing could be farther from the truth. Yet on these grossly mistaken ideas are based the shame and terror so many of us feel when we are faced with the thought or the presence of mental illness.

People will talk about their physical ailments without the slightest inhibition. They will bore listeners to distraction with detailed and repeated accounts of their operations and accidents. But let the illness or injury be mental and they will go to absurd lengths to hide it, concocting elaborate lies and evasions to keep it from being known.

Perhaps this is both the cause and the effect of our not knowing how much mental illness there is in the land. One out of every five families in the United States at some time has one of its members in a mental hospital. There are today more than 700,000 patients in mental hospitals in the United States—more than the total of patients hospitalized for all other causes combined! We have more hospitalized cases of dementia praecox—the mental disorder that strikes youth in its teens and early 20's—than of tuberculosis!

Severe mental illness, like severe physical illness, is a misfortune. But it is no greater tragedy and no more disgraceful than is a case of paralysis, for instance. The man with a disordered mind can no more help it, is no more to blame for his condition, than is the man with a disordered body. And if the two are service veterans, one is just as much a war casualty, just as much a hero, as the other.

The truth about N-P's

The war has made it imperative that we bring our ideas on this subject quickly up to date. Otherwise thousands of returning servicemen and their families will undergo needless torments of mind and soul. For the war is ripping our unawareness to shreds; it is uncovering the incidence of mental and emotional disorders at a pace and in a volume that cannot be ignored.

By the end of 1944 one and a quarter million men between the ages of eighteen and thirty-eight had been rejected by induction board examiners for some mental or emotional condition that made them unfit for military service. Three hundred and fifty thousand more had been discharged from the services for the same reason, and these discharges were continuing at the rate of some thirty thousand each month. Nearly one half (forty-five per cent) of all medical discharges from the armed forces are for some mental or emotional disorder.

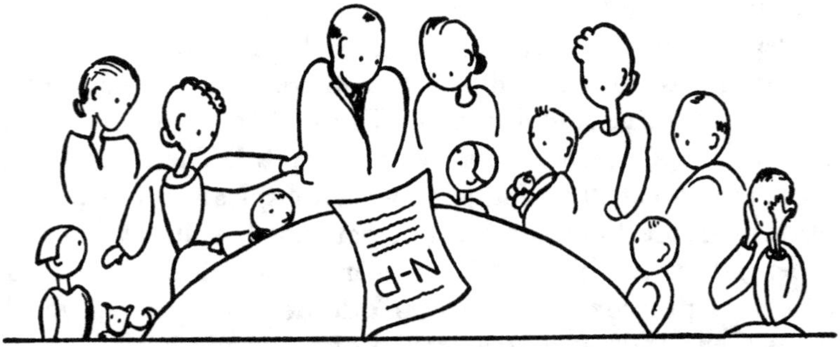

What does it mean?

From time to time the military authorities have changed the word or phrase used to designate these discharges, but the first one chosen is the one that has got into conversation and print, and it clings to all the later equivalents. It is the word *neuropsychiatric,* popularly shortened to N-P.

Many of the veterans who have received N-P discharges do not know exactly why. All they have is a long word they do not know the meaning of, plus a vague notion that it has something to do with their minds or their behavior. So they worry about it. And so do their families. The womenfolk are tearful and anxious, wondering whether their serviceman is losing his mind, or they are ashamed, thinking the N-P label means that he has been a coward, afraid to fight, or that he has a weak character, or that his intelligence is below par.

A neuropsychiatric discharge is a discharge for some mental or emotional disability, but such disabilities are of all sorts and degrees, just as physical disabilities are. If you were told that a veteran had been discharged for a physical disability, you would not know whether he had a severe paralysis like Joe's, a missing arm like Dick's, or something as innocuous as flat feet or a punctured eardrum. These last two may be physical disabilities for military service, but they certainly do not prejudice one's success in civilian activities.

Similarly a discharge for mental disability tells nothing about the kind or the seriousness of the cause. The disability may be anything from faintness at the sight of blood to a severe case of insanity. Actually it means insanity in relatively few cases, and these cases will almost certainly be kept in the hospital.

So an N-P discharge of itself is nothing to be upset about. If you are physically ill, you do not assume that your life is in danger just because some people who are physically ill have serious diseases. In the same way, if your serviceman comes home with an N-P discharge, don't jump to the conclusion that he is in desperate mental straits just because some N-P cases are. At a time when he needs understanding and encouragement to restore his self-confidence and overcome his worries and fears, don't deal him the blow of showing suspicion or shame in your face or your manner.

Many N-P's have only what the layman would call a case of nerves; they are tense and jumpy, can't sleep, have bad dreams about their army experiences, have no pep and tire easily, and so on. They will probably need only a few months of reconditioning to put them on their feet again.

Others are subject to headaches, nervous indigestion, high blood pressure, heart palpitations, diarrhea, dizziness — all conditions that can be brought on by nervous tension and too much worrying about problems big and little. The men probably had these difficulties in some degree before they entered the army. Which of us does not number among his acquaintances several civilians who suffer from similar ailments—business executives who munch soda mint tablets while they dictate their letters and contracts, university professors who punctuate their daily duties with doses of baking soda from the box or bottle in their desk drawer, newspapermen who can't sleep without large doses of sedative? But in the army there can be no baking soda in the K rations, and battle with the enemy cannot wait until GI Joe mixes himself a dose of bromide. So he must be discharged as unfit for military service.

The N-P is not a weakling, not a coward, and not a slacker. He is much more likely to be the overconscientious kind of person who cannot shirk, who works too tensely and too hard, who cannot take things easily or run away from his job; that is why he has broken down. He is not lacking in will power. His mental illness is no more his fault than if he had got a bullet wound or a case of malaria, and it is no more a reflection on his character or that of his family.

Mental illness

We have been using the terms *mental* illness, *mental* disorder, *mental* disability, because they seem the simplest and the commonest. Other writers prefer to use other names, such as *nervous* illness, or *emotional* disability, or *psychiatric* condition, or *personality* disorder. The name used does not matter; the important thing is the state or condition that all these terms are applied to. What is this mental, emotional, or nervous condition we are talking about?

We can clear one common confusion out of the way immediately. It is *not* feeblemindedness. That is a condition of mental deficiency, in which the person is born without a normal mental equipment or loses it because of disease or injury in childhood. His mental powers never attain their full development. He remains a child in mind though he becomes an adult in body.

Such persons are called idiots, imbeciles, or morons according to the mental age at which their minds stop growing. Some of them never progress beyond the mental status of an infant, never learning to talk and requiring throughout their lives the care usually given to babies. Others can learn to read and write but not to think or act with sufficient intelligence to earn their living or to take a responsible place in society.

When these adult children cannot be accommodated in the special state schools maintained for them, they are sometimes cared for in state hospitals for the mentally ill. This may in part account for the layman's confusion of mental deficiency with mental illness.

Mental illness is a disorder or loss of function occurring in a mind that was normal, perhaps even exceptional. The trouble may be minor and temporary, or it may be serious and prolonged, but while it lasts the patient's mind does not function at its full capacity or efficiency.

This is one of the mistakes Sarah is making in her thinking about Ted. She cannot believe that anything could have happened to Ted's mind because he always did so well in his studies. She does not understand that mental breakdowns can come to persons of brilliant intelligence. She is thinking of the mind as only the ability to learn.

Just what do we mean by the word *mind?* Webster's dictionary gives twelve meanings in general usage, and the psychologists could add a few more technical meanings. To nine in ten laymen, however, the word *mind* probably means first the intellect—the thinking, reasoning faculty of man. Yet mental illness often has little or nothing to do with the intellect as such.

Everyman's equipment for meeting the manifold demands of life includes his physical body, with all its bones, muscles, blood vessels, and internal organs; his individual allotment of the faculty we call intelligence; and his set of emotions or feelings. No one of these three is an isolated unit, functioning alone. They are closely and intricately intermeshed, so that anything wrong with any one of them is very likely to throw the others out of gear. Together they constitute the total person or personality, and when they are working together in harmony and proper balance, the individual is well adjusted, at his peak of happiness and efficiency in meeting the problems of life. The apparatus whose function is to maintain this harmony and balance, the automatic pilot or control, is the nervous system centering in the brain.

This being the case, when we oppose physical illness (of the body) to mental illness (of the mind), we must include in our concept of the mind not only the intellect but also the emotions and all the complex mechanism of adjustment and balance that operates through the nervous system. This is why some experts prefer to call the illness nervous, emotional, or of the personality—to get away from the idea that it is a disorder only of the intellect.

Perhaps *psychiatric* illness is the best term, since, being a newer word without all the connotations that usage has attached to the others, it can be defined for our purposes as any impairment or derangement of the intellectual, emotional, or nervous equipment with which we make our way through life.

Such psychiatric or mental illness may be caused by actual physical injury or disease in the nervous system or the brain. It is then called an *organic* mental disorder. The delirium caused by a high fever or by acute alcoholism is such a mental illness. So is the loss of memory resulting from a blow on the head, and the deterioration or decay of mental faculties that sometimes occurs in old age (senile dementia) or in an advanced stage of syphilis (general paresis).

In many cases of psychiatric disorder, however, no such physical cause can be discovered. Doctors are inclined to think of these cases as psychological in origin. The illness is just as real, but its cause is some failure in the functioning of the mind, in the way it works, rather than in any defect or damage of the physical structure. It is these *functional* psychiatric disorders with which we are concerned in this chapter and the next.

All men are not equal

Just how these functional disorders come about is not yet fully known. After all, psychiatry is the youngest of the medical specialties, and psychology, the science of the mind, is not much older. If doctors and medical scientists with a much longer history have not yet uncovered the causes and processes of all physical disease, it is no cause for surprise or suspicion that the experts do not know everything about mental illness and do not agree on all its aspects.

One of the matters on which they do not agree is the relative roles of heredity and environment. We can safely say, however, that just as some persons are born with less physical stamina than others, with less resistance to disease, less physical strength and endurance, so some are born with less mental and emotional stamina, less resistance to the strain of life's crises and conflicts. Just as one may be born with some inherited weakness in the kidneys or the lungs or the heart that predisposes him to disease in that organ, so perhaps one may come into the world with some weakness in his nervous or emotional system that predisposes him to a breakdown when the going gets too tough.

But the individual's inherited constitution is not the whole answer. Suppose two boys are born with similar constitutional predispositions toward tuberculosis. One grows up in a tenement district, gets little sunlight and fresh air, eats improper food and not enough of it, must help to support the family by selling newspapers on the street corner in all kinds of weather without enough warm clothing. The other spends a well-regulated childhood on a farm, plays out of doors much of the time, has enough clothing to meet any change in the weather, eats all the milk, eggs, meat, and vegetables he wants. Bring these two boys together in later life in identical conditions of exposure. The first will almost certainly contract tuberculosis, the second probably will not. Whatever the physical constitution one is born with, it can be strengthened or weakened by the environment in which he grows up.

One's mental constitution too may be weakened or

strengthened by the circumstances of one's upbringing. From babyhood on, everyman's life is a constant problem of adjustment: to his own body and the strange new world around him, to others in his family, to his playmates at school and his parents' grownup friends, to his business associates or fellow workers. He must adapt himself also to all the social conventions and cultural customs of his society, and to a host of situations and happenings that bring him by turn failure and success, responsibility and danger, grief and disappointment, hate and love, fear and anger.

How will he react to other people? With suspicion of their motives and critical condemnation of their actions, or with friendly tolerance of their different ways, sure of their good intentions? Will he fly into a rage over every minor disappointment, or will he accept frustration with a philosophic shrug of the shoulders, knowing it to be the common lot of man? Will he make decisions quickly and press forward without futile regrets, or will he fret himself sick over even the choice of a new suit and be forever crying over spilled milk? Will he shoulder responsibility with confidence or with nerves tense from fear of failure? Or will he shirk responsibility entirely, even for his own decisions?

These and the scores of other habit patterns that make up one's personality are formed in childhood and adolescence. A child may acquire them from precept, of course. What his parents teach him about moral and ethical behavior becomes his conscience or lack of it in adult life.

But he may also acquire them by imitation. If his parents face new experiences and unexpected crises with confidence and serenity, his muscles and nerves will tend to copy their pattern of relaxed strength. But if his mother is a bundle of nerves, meeting even a thunderstorm with apprehension, she need not say a word; he will learn by imitation her pattern of nervous tension when the thunder and lightning appear.

A child may also, and most effectively perhaps, acquire his methods of response by experience. Suppose he wants to go outside to play. His mother says no. Instantly and automatically all his inner resources are mobilized to find a way to avoid this thwarting of his wishes. He tries coaxing and whining. If his mother gives in, fine. If not, he may try a temper tantrum. If that doesn't work, he may turn to sulking, or pinching sister, or tormenting the cat, or otherwise making a nuisance of himself. When he hits upon a method that gets him what he wants, he will remember and use it again. And as long as it continues to work, he will continue to use it, until it becomes his habitual way of dealing with frustration of any kind.

As he grows to manhood, the form of his temper tantrum, sulking, or tormenting may change, but the basic method will remain the same. An adult in a business office can hardly kick, scream, and hold his breath, but he may curse till the air is blue and pound the desk top till the inkwell jumps. The second piece of behavior is as much a temper tantrum as the first.

For good mental health, the personality patterns acquired in these ways — by precept, imitation, and experience — must be numerous, flexible, and sound enough to carry the individual with reasonable efficiency and comfort through the whole gamut of life's problems. If his patterns are few, rigid, or unacceptable to society, he may not be able to surmount his mental conflicts.

As this implies, heredity and upbringing do not alone determine the incidence of mental illness. Their results depend

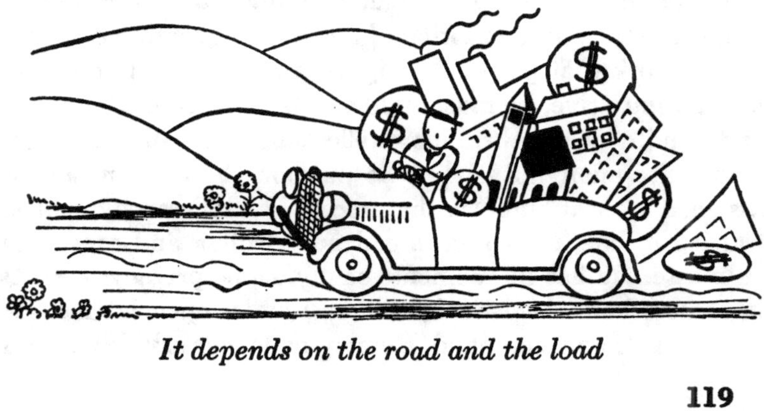

It depends on the road and the load

on what demands life makes of the individual. They merely set the limits of his endurance, determine the amount and the kind of stress he can take without breaking down. His heredity may be bad, his upbringing faulty, yet if fate gives him or he makes for himself a smooth, even course, without turnings too sudden or hills too high, he may live out his days without illness.

On the other hand, in the face of drastic changes, multiplying problems, and mounting strain, every person, whatever his heredity and environment, has a breaking point. Just as the strongest physical constitution will give way to exhaustion and disease if the load carried is too heavy or the exposure to cold and snow too long, so the strongest mental and emotional constitution will crack if the going gets too tough or the strain lasts too long.

From civilian to soldier

Few men in an ordinary lifetime are called upon to make the sudden and extensive readjustment that modern warfare demands. Its methods and principles are so different from American ways in peacetime that they constitute a shift into reverse which would strip the gears of the best man-made machine. It is not to be wondered at that some men find it beyond their powers.

The change from civilian to soldier uproots a man from his home, his family and friends, his customary activities, and sets him down in unfamiliar surroundings, among strangers, to live a totally different kind of life. After a training in school and at work that places the highest premium on individuality and initiative, he must suddenly try to lose his indentity and hand over to others his intellect and his will. He begins to acquire anonymity when he puts on the uniform and is assigned a serial number; the process is furthered by endless waiting in line, marching in cadence, drilling and exercising en masse. He has no moments of inviolable privacy; he eats in a mess hall, sleeps in barracks, uses an open latrine. He lives by rule and command. He may no longer ask, What do I think? What do I feel? What do I want? He must ask instead, What are the orders?

This loss of freedom to arrange the details of one's own life may bring to light hitherto unsuspected or unrecognized difficulties. This is strikingly illustrated in a case history reported by Dr. George K. Pratt in his very helpful book *Soldier to Civilian*.

Luigi Santozzi was a finicky eater. He was addicted to food fads and was constantly experimenting with some new diet, testing out its possible effects on his stomach. Having driven his mother to revolt with his demands for special cooking, he began frequenting special restaurants, changing from one to another as he got bored with each new diet in turn.

Luigi had other peculiarities too. For instance, he had developed an aversion to woolen clothing. Not because the wool made him break out in a rash or had any other physical effect on him, but because he decided that it was unhealthy for him. Even in wintertime he went to extreme lengths to find suits and coats without wool.

Luigi's feelings were easily and often hurt. If a salesman spoke sharply to him or the waitress at his restaurant of the moment did not give him the service he thought he ought to have, he would impulsively leave the store or restaurant and go elsewhere. In the same way he was always changing jobs. When anything in one job didn't please him — the surroundings, the attitude of the foreman, the personality of the worker next to him — he simply quit and found another job. This happened so often that he did not remain in any one place long enough for his peculiarities to become conspicuous.

On the whole Luigi had a pretty thoroughly disordered personality, but as long as he could shape his own life he got on all right — not very comfortably or conveniently by other folks' standards, but without any serious disturbance. His family and friends were probably amused at all his queer notions, but they did not consider him mentally ill.

Then Luigi became a seaman in the navy. And here he could no longer arrange his life in accordance with his sick ideas. He did for a time manage to avoid eating in the mess hall, claiming the navy food upset his stomach and getting along on the things he could buy at the canteen. But he had to wear his navy blues despite their wool content, and he could not quit when the commanding officer spoke sharply to him.

Under these limitations his sickness showed up. He grew depressed, tense, and anxious, and when his duties took him below deck to work in a shut-in place he got so panicky that once he ran around screaming in terror. It was finally clear that he could not work efficiently or be depended on in a crisis; so he was given an N-P discharge. Back in civilian life, free once more to arrange his own life, he may get along without a breakdown. But he would be wise to see a psychiatrist who could give him some understanding of his behavior.

He fought on two fronts

The new soldier must also reverse some of his established ideas of right and wrong. He has been taught to respect honesty, decency, fair play, and sportsmanship, to take thought for and uphold the rights of others, to respect the dignity of human life in any form.

Now almost overnight he must become an efficient killer. using any form of trickery, deceit, or cunning that will give him an advantage over the enemy. Not only must he forget that the individual enemy is a human being like himself, but if the strain of warfare is not to get him down, he must think of his fellow soldiers not as persons but as military expendables. He must do his best to callous his emotions, to become immune to the personal tragedies of war.

This adjustment seems to have been Ted's principal stumbling block. Sarah can see no significance in the things Ted said and did when he was home on furlough, but they are suggestive of the trouble ahead. The very qualities that made Ted a good son, good neighbor, and good teacher have almost certainly aggravated the difficulty of his adjustment to military life.

He was a quiet, studious young man, accustomed to nothing more upsetting than the high-spirited pranks of youngsters in the classroom. He would not take readily to the constant activity, the hubbub, the lack of privacy in army life. But he might have got used to this in time. What it seems he could not do is to forget that men are men. Those youthful prisoners he had to guard were not just objects to him; they were boys like the ones he had taught in high school. He just couldn't shoot at them.

This would not have been disastrous perhaps if Ted had been able to say to himself: "All right, I won't shoot at them. I know I must obey orders or be punished. But these orders are cruel and unfair. I won't obey them; I'll take the punishment instead." Had Ted been able to reason the matter out with himself like this, there would have been no wearing conflict in his mind. But he could not make such a clear-cut decision because it runs counter to another well-established pattern in his personality. He has always been obedient to those in authority over him. He likes people and needs to have them like him, and he has learned from childhood to secure this liking by doing what others ask of him. He has not learned to take their disapproval without distress when he is doing what he thinks is right.

So these two patterns of behavior staged a devastating tug of war in Ted's mind. The first won out, but the second was too strong for Ted to forget it when the incident was over.

If Ted couldn't shoot to discipline his prisoners, it is not likely that he could face calmly the prospect of shooting or bayoneting to kill. He probably refused to admit this even to himself, but his insistence to his mother that he wouldn't mind meeting the enemy suggests that the idea was troubling him. He was afraid he would not be able to kill, and he was afraid he would be called a coward if he didn't. This second fear was expressing itself perhaps in his fixed aversion to yellow and in his disinclination to meet and talk with old friends.

These conflicts in Ted's mind, conflicts he could not resolve, turned his mind into a battleground as destructive of mental health as any combat field could be. In the end they caused him to break down.

Too little and too late

Adjustments to military service are not equally difficult for all men, of course. The more sensitive and imaginative the person and the greater his sense of human values, the less likely he is to accept violence casually or to live comfortably with danger and in the presence of death. The man accustomed to do his daily work under orders will exchange his foreman or superintendent for an army sergeant without too much trouble. But for the executive who is used to giving orders, or for the artist who lives by emphasizing his individuality, the required conformity to a mass pattern may be impossible.

Even leaving home is not so difficult for some as for others. Some men may even find it a relief to get away: for instance, the man who, unconsciously perhaps, has been longing for freedom from a wife he has ceased to love; or the unmarried man whose sense of filial duty has kept him at the side of a widowed mother much against his will; or the boy who is chafing under too much parental domination. For them military service is a way of leaving behind an unpleasant situation without incurring legal penalties or social disapproval. They may after a time find army or navy life as little to their liking as the old, but their sense of release at the moment of change will lessen their problem of adjustment.

On the other hand, breaking home ties may be difficult beyond endurance for the boy or man whose mother has never let him make a decision of his own, spend so much as a single night away from home, or in any way live his own life; for the man who has centered his entire emotional life on his wife and children, having few friends and almost no social life or recreation outside his home; or for the man whose range of experience is too limited to make him aware or tolerant of other attitudes and ways than those he has been taught.

Russell was this third sort of man. He grew up in a small

town, one of two children in a devoutly religious family. His parents' highly moral standards of behavior were strictly enforced upon the children. Disobedience in any degree brought immediate and severe punishment. The use of liquor in any amount was forbidden as a moral evil, and Russell learned, mostly from their tight-lipped silences, what his parents thought of men who got drunk. In somewhat the same indirect but nonetheless effective way he learned what they and the community in general considered the limits of propriety in relations between the sexes.

Russell grew to manhood without any notion that these standards of behavior are not accepted, or at least adhered to, by all good people. So in the army he was at first outraged and then bewildered by the words and actions of his fellow soldiers. They accepted as a matter of course things he considered sinful and they laughed at what they called his screwy notions. He had to admit they were goodhearted and generous, most of them; they would go to any amount of trouble to help a fellow out of a jam. And he very much needed their companionship. He was finding it hard going in the army because he worried so about everything—afraid he'd break a rule or fail to carry out an order. The fellows laughed at him for this too; they didn't know how strong a part of his personality was the habit of exact obedience.

One night Russell's loneliness overcame his scruples and he went with a couple of the fellows into town on a three-hour pass. They teased and prodded him into taking a drink. He didn't much like the taste of it but it didn't seem to affect him in any way. So he had another and began to join in the chaffing between his buddies and a couple of girls at the bar.

Russell woke up the next morning in a hotel room with a strange girl. When he understood what had happened, that he had overstayed his leave and had slept with this girl, he suddenly began to tremble with fear, and by the time he arrived back at camp he was hysterical. Although he got over this immediate illness, he could not forget what had happened. He would suddenly break out in a cold sweat at the very thought of his mother and his sweetheart. What would happen if they should hear what he had done? He brooded over this in the daytime and worried over it even in his sleep, until he became ill and had to be hospitalized. He was then given an N-P discharge.

Russell's trouble lay in his few and rigid patterns of behavior. Nothing in his background training had given him tolerance or understanding of human frailty in himself or in others. And unfortunately an experience too drastic for him to handle came to him before he could gain such understanding for himself through observation of different kinds of human behavior.

The strain is not the same

Although a great many psychiatric breakdowns occur, like Ted's and Russell's, during the period of training, most men manage by one device or another to get through this period of adjustment. They get used to the goldfish-bowl life, learn to take the sergeant's loud reprimands and the other men's rough kidding. They are able somehow to reconcile their conflicts and to rationalize the new behavior required of them satisfactorily enough to retain their emotional balance. So they go on to combat overseas.

In combat the soldier may run into experiences so violent and so shattering that even the soundest minds cannot take too large a dose without severe reaction. But why is it that of a group of men going through the same battle experience some come back with disabling emotional upsets while the others, though tired, are fit for further duty?

We say they go through the same experience, but do they? For one it may be the first taste of combat, for others the tenth or twentieth; the strain is not the same. Perhaps one sets out on a mission over Tokyo after a sleepless night brought on by a letter from home telling him his sweetheart has married another man. The strain of whatever happens will be greater for him than for his buddies who know that all is well back home.

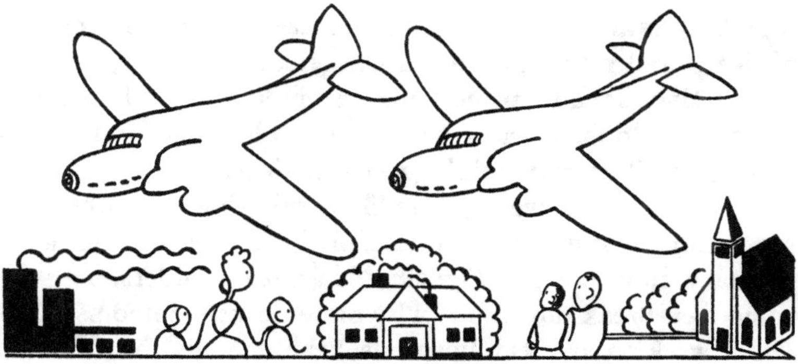

The strain is not the same

Or perhaps two men in battle see the man ahead blown to pieces by an exploding mine. For one the experience is intolerable because the man is his best friend; for the other, bad as the sight is, it remains impersonal because he did not know the man. The two do not go through the same experience, because the strain of any situation depends upon inner as well as outer circumstances.

For this reason some men may break in combat sooner than others, but every man will reach the limit of his endurance if the missions or battles are too many without rest, if the sights are too terrible, if the accompanying exhaustion, exposure, and discomfort are too severe or too long continued. There will come a time when his mind and nerves cannot take one minute more of it.

Ernie Pyle reached this point and described it in the last column he wrote before coming home from Europe for an imperative rest: "I am leaving for only one reason—because I have just got to stop. . . . I've had all I can take for a while . . . I've been immersed in it for too long. My spirit is wobbly and my mind confused. The hurt has finally become too great. All of a sudden it seemed to me that if I heard one more shot or saw one more dead man, I would go off my nut. And if I had to write one more column, I'd collapse."

The quality of mind and spirit that made Ernie Pyle America's favorite war correspondent—his ability to see and report the war in individual, human terms — made every bit of death and mutilation he saw a personal tragedy, and the cumulative shock to his nervous system finally got him down. He just couldn't consider these soldiers he knew and understood so well as mere military expendables.

When one reads war reports like Ernie Pyle's, or when one sees glimpses of battle conditions in the newsreels or in documentary films like *The Fighting Lady*, one wonders, not why some men break down, but why more do not. Some psychiatrists working in field hospitals near enough the front to know what combat conditions are like have come to wonder whether the men who break are not the really normal ones.

The father who failed

Yet some civilians to whom the war has brought no danger and little discomfort call these men weaklings. They act like Smoky's father. As the pilot of a giant bomber, Smoky flew mission after mission over Germany, until all but one other of his outfit had been killed, until his face was gaunt, his body thin, from the strain.

Then one day he had to watch while a German fighter got the bomber ahead of him, the bomber piloted by a guy he had known and liked since their first days of training together. Helplessly Smoky watched the bomber plummet downward, leaving a twisted trail of black smoke behind. He strained his eyes to see the parachute that might mean his friend was getting free of the doomed plane. But no parachute appeared.

Smoky couldn't forget that sight, and he went around tense and sleepless for days. Then his flight surgeon recommended a rest, which turned finally into an N-P discharge. Smoky took this hard until the doctor explained it to him: "You've been going through dangers you'd never have had to face as a civilian. And you've reached your limit. Every man has one, you know. Your nerves just won't stand any more action. Back home with your family again, you'll be all right."

Smoky felt better after this, except on one point. All the way across the Atlantic to the hospital in New York he worried about how his folks would take his cracking up. What would his dad say? When he spoke about this to the man in the next bed, the man said, "Listen, kid. Quit worrying. You've gone through hell. Now you need some help. Your dad will understand."

But his dad didn't. When he came to the hospital he was cold and hard. "I'm ashamed of you," he said to Smoky. "I didn't think you would do a thing like this."

Smoky would have been all right, as the doctor said, with some understanding and encouragement. But his father didn't give them to him. So he's still in the mental hospital, fighting his sick nerves alone.

Preventive measures

Experience, especially in World War I, has made the military authorities increasingly aware of the importance of the fact that all men are not equally suited to military duty, just as all men are not equally suited to mountain climbing or to scientific exploration in remote wildernesses.

When war comes the armed forces have a tremendous job to do, and they must do it with all possible speed. They cannot afford the time and effort required to deal with those who cannot fit in reasonably well after a period of adjustment. Besides, such men may prove a real danger to the lives and morale of their fellows at a critical point in battle or in the close quarters of a ship at sea or the closer quarters of a plane in the air.

So a psychiatric examination has been added to the physical screening at induction centers. Under the circumstances this can be only a brief and superficial questioning, but even so it eliminates about one in eight of those who take it. Rejection for psychiatric reasons as for physical disability is a preventive measure for the individual as well as for the armed services; it saves a man from a situation he is not equal to and so from a possible breakdown.

But here again misunderstanding and ignorance may work their harm. The man rejected for defective eyesight or underweight may regret it, but neither he nor anyone else considers it cause for reproach. The man rejected for some psychiatric disability, however, is likely to worry about it, to be depressed and ashamed, and to make up a story about some invisible physical defect to conceal the facts from his friends.

The verdict of the induction examiner does not change the man in any way. If he has been getting along all right before, there is no reason why he should not continue to do so. Perhaps his trouble is fainting at the sight of blood. Obviously this disqualifies him from military service, but it hardly affects his civilian success unless he tries to become a butcher or a surgeon.

It may be that his condition is something he has not suspected and that he should see a doctor about — as should the man for whom the examination has brought to light an incipient case of tuberculosis he did not know he had. But it may just as well be that the trouble is too slight to bother about. We repeat: Military standards differ from civilian requirements, so that unfitness for military service does not necessarily mean unfitness for a good civilian job.

Within the armed services the facilities for psychiatric treatment and measures to prevent possible breakdowns were spotty and inadequate in the early stages of the war, but they steadily improved in several directions. More attention was given to morale and there was increasing appreciation of the fact that sustaining morale requires something more than keeping the boys entertained. Aware of the problems and conflicts that may precipitate breakdowns, the services tried to prepare their men against the things that might trouble them.

The reasons for military discipline were explained to them: It is imperative that they learn to obey orders without question because in battle others' lives and their own may depend on their doing so, and the very disinclination of raw recruits to do so makes it necessary that their training be thorough and severe. It was explained to them that bravery and heroism do not mean the absence of fear, that all men are afraid before and during combat, that being afraid does not make a man a coward.

Because the man who fights best under incredible hardship and who is most nearly impervious to breakdown is the man who knows why he is fighting, the services have given a good deal of time to lectures, discussions, and motion pictures on "Why We Fight," in the hope of showing the men why it suddenly became, in the opinion of most of us, necessary and right to kill.

The whole training program has been aimed at preparing the men for every foreseeable contingency in battle, so their reactions to danger may be almost automatic and they will not have to face unknown situations and make vital decisions in a time of terror.

The psychiatric staff was enlarged and reorganized; mental hygiene clinics were set up in training camps, and certain noncommissioned officers who lived with the men were trained to spot the early signs of nervous and emotional disturbances. Men in whom these signs appeared were referred at once to the nearest medical officer or psychiatric counselor in an effort to discover the cause of their trouble and straighten it out before it reached the breakdown stage.

When illness comes in spite of these preventive measures, the goal is to start treatment as quickly as possible. Psychiatrists have learned that the longer mental symptoms are allowed to go on unchecked, the more likely they are to become fixed as habits and the more difficult it is to get rid of them. Unfortunately the shortage of trained psychiatrists and the conditions of combat make it impossible always to achieve the ideal of immediate treatment, speedy recovery, and return to duty. When this result is not obtained, the men are sent to special hospitals for treatment, those from overseas being returned to the United States.

The care and treatment provided in these special hospitals have been expanded and improved, especially during 1945, so that everything possible is done to make the men fit again for a good civilian life before discharging them.

Not all the same

The breakdowns we have been discussing are not equally severe or of the same type. They are of two general kinds, each of which may occur in varying degrees of severity. The first kind is characterized by such symptoms as hallucinations, delusions, stupor, wild elation, and so on. Doctors call this kind of breakdown a psychosis, and what the layman calls insanity belongs in this class.

The second kind is characterized by *exaggerated* anxiety, fear, worry, depression, and such physical symptoms as these mental upsets may produce: headaches, stomach pain, heart palpitations, and the like. This kind of breakdown the doctors call neurosis, or preferably psychoneurosis. The layman, when he recognizes it, thinks of it as a bad case of nerves or nervous jitters.

Psychosis and *psychoneurosis*. If these words seem formidable, it is only because they are still unfamiliar. They are no longer or harder than *tuberculosis, tonsilitis,* or *appendicitis,* and they are no more mysterious or dreadful. Since they are appearing more and more frequently in talk and in print, making clear what they mean will help to dispel the undeserved stigma attached to them. Evading the use of them only gives them an importance they do not deserve—and is an insult to the layman's intelligence besides.

Whole volumes have been written about these two forms of mental illness, so what we can tell you here is only a brief and general outline.

Doctors cannot in all stages or cases tell these two kinds of illness apart—just as a few years ago they could not always be sure whether a patient's pain in the abdomen came from appendicitis or from gallstones. But *in clearly defined cases* psychosis and psychoneurosis are two fairly distinct kinds of mental disorder, and the major difference between them is this: In psychosis the patient in some degree loses touch with the real world around him; he talks and acts "queer." He lives in an inner dream world of his own and so behaves at variance with the world familiar to the rest of us. And in most cases he is not aware of this; he does not know that he is ill, that his thoughts and acts are irrational.

In psychoneurosis the patient seldom if ever loses his touch with reality. His difficulties in adjusting to the world may be far greater than those of the average person, but they are the difficulties all of us have. He knows, or can be made to know, that his fears and worries are irrational, although knowing this will not alone dispel them. In psychoneurosis, too, only a part of the individual's personality is affected; a woman with a neurotic (that is, an exaggerated) fear of mice is quite normal when there are no mice around. In most cases of psychosis, on the other hand, much more of the personality is involved.

This does not mean that psychoneurosis is a mild form of mental illness likely to develop into the severe form of psychosis. The relationship between them is perhaps more nearly like that between chicken pox and smallpox. In general, chicken pox is the milder disease, smallpox the more severe, but one may have a bad case of chicken pox or a mild case of smallpox. And chicken pox does not become smallpox.

In somewhat the same way a psychoneurosis rarely crosses the line into psychosis. The psychoneurotic may be more handicapped for effective living than the person with a mild psychosis, but his illness remains psychoneurosis. Why some people break down psychotically and others psychoneurotically is one of the aspects of mental illness that doctors do not yet understand.

Among both civilians and servicemen there are many, many more cases of psychoneurosis than of psychosis. Only ten in one hundred of those discharged from the armed forces for mental and emotional disorders are psychotic. It is with these few that the remainder of this chapter deals.

Outward signs

The diagnosis of psychiatric illness is the province of the doctor. The layman has no more business trying it on his own than he would have diagnosing pneumonia or diphtheria for himself. Nonetheless one has to know some of the obvious symptoms of physical illness in order to know when to call the doctor. For the same purpose, and also to make clearer the difference between psychosis and psychoneurosis, we shall try to give here a brief description of some of the most noticeable symptoms of psychosis.

However, if you are one of those persons who are sure they have every illness they hear or read about, from gallstones to housemaid's knee, you had better read the warning given on page 136 before reading this section.

Hallucinations are one of the symptoms of psychosis. These may be roughly defined as false sense impressions. The patient sees things that are not there for another's eyes, or he hears voices that are audible to no one else, or he smells odors that do not exist, or tastes poison in his food when it is not present. Hearing nonexistent voices is the most common form of hallucination.

Delusions are closely related to hallucinations and sometimes accompany them. Delusions are false beliefs instead of false sensations. Instead of seeing objects that do not exist, the patient believes he is a king, or an inventor, or a millionaire, or that someone is trying to kill him—*when none of these is true*. In another kind of delusion, he thinks that everything anyone around him does is intended somehow to injure him. He has "delusions of persecution."

The most striking feature of a delusion is its fixity; the patient can in no way be argued out of it or made to see that it isn't true. For this reason delusions are sometimes called fixed ideas.

Sometimes the patient's false beliefs and his conduct are entirely divorced. For instance, the man who believes he is the King of England may be quite content to mop the floors or mow the lawn, and the millionaire will beg for a bit of tobacco, neither of them recognizing any inconsistency in his acts. On the other hand, a person with delusions of persecution may try to attack his imagined enemies and thus become a source of danger in the community.

Another psychotic symptom is extreme excitement *without adequate cause and entirely out of keeping with the patient's real circumstances.* Such a person is in a state of constant overactivity, commencing a new occupation at every minute and immediately abandoning it for another. He talks rapidly and incessantly, and often quite incoherently; words or phrases are distorted in meaning or misplaced or omitted altogether, making what he says a meaningless word salad. His abnormal elation may change to furious anger at the slightest provocation, and in extreme cases he may become violently combative.

Extreme depression is the opposite of such excitement. *Without observable cause* the patient slows down mentally in all his speech and actions. He thinks with difficulty, talks slowly and hesitantly if at all. He is thoroughly unhappy and miserable, despondent *out of all proportion to his circumstances.* He must be constantly guarded against suicide.

In another psychotic state the patient is neither excited nor depressed but is absolutely indifferent, without any apparent interests or desires. He may sit for hours on end with an expressionless face, his head hanging, making no attempt to do anything, taking no notice of what goes on around him. If he pays any attention to questions, he answers only in monosyllables. If the doctor can stimulate him out of his stupor it becomes clear that he can observe, remember, think, and talk perfectly well. His trouble is not a loss of intellect but a profound emotional apathy.

Stereotyped actions are another symptom of psychosis. The patient carries out some purposeless action with monotonous repetition day in and day out for months on end perhaps. All his energy and attention are absorbed by it, so that he has no other interest and does nothing else. These actions may vary from a simple rhythmical movement of the hands or the head to elaborate motions that suggest the manipulations of a skilled craftsman. Or the stereotyped activity may be the monotonous repetition of a meaningless phrase or sentence.

A psychosis is not limited to any one of these symptoms, nor need they all be present. Along with others less obvious they appear in varying combinations. Just as a certain pattern of physical symptoms tells the doctor that his patient has bronchitis or diphtheria or pneumonia, so the pattern of the mental symptoms tells him that the man is suffering from schizophrenia or paranoia or a manic-depressive psychosis. These three terms that appear so frequently nowadays in newspapers, magazines, and even novels are the names of three kinds of psychosis.

Warning: Seek not or ye shall find

Do not go around looking for these symptoms in yourself and all your friends, because if you do you will surely think you have found them; *they all exist in some degree in the perfectly normal mind.* This cannot be overemphasized. Suspiciousness, daydreaming in a fantasy world of one's own,

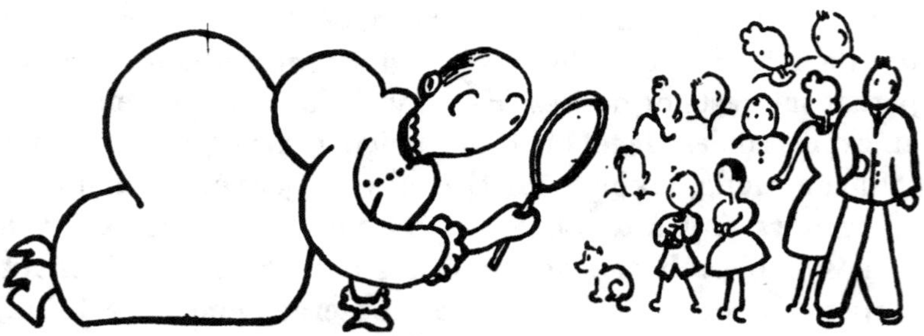

A symptom hunter

inexplicable changes of mood from happy well-being to gloomy despair, periods of emotional fatigue when nothing seems worth the energy it takes, a tendency to repeat futile little gestures or motions—all these things are commonly present in an entirely healthy mind. It is only when such habits or characteristics take over the mind to the exclusion of reality that they become abnormal.

A serious or sudden *change* of behavior is the significant sign of oncoming mental illness. But again, this does not mean you should become alarmed every time a member of your family does something peculiar or unusual. It is not abnormal for your son to be depressed for a while after his girl has jilted him. Nor is your husband suffering delusions of persecution if he comes home from a hard day at the office and says he'd like to wring the boss's neck.

You must use your common sense. You do not worry every time one of your family gets a headache or a slight cold, but if he cannot go to work because he is feverish or in pain, or if you think he may be a danger to the community because he has a skin rash, you send for the doctor. Send for him too if anyone in your family becomes unable to carry on his daily activities because he sits around brooding for hours on end, or if he begins acting silly, grinning and laughing foolishly without any reason, or if he develops queer notions about poison in his food or little men in his bedroom, or if he suddenly becomes destructive, tearing up the bedclothes or the neighbor's picket fence.

If something like this should happen, don't just think of your relative as wicked, or stubborn, or lazy. Don't scold or argue or reprove; don't "tell him where to get off," urge him to "snap out of it," or wish he'd get religion so he'd be less ornery and malicious. These methods won't work because he can't help his actions, any more than he could stop having a fever just by exercising his will power. He is sick. He doesn't need a lawyer, a minister, or a policeman; he needs a doctor. And the sooner the doctor is called the better.

Don't wait, thinking the symptoms will clear up after a while; they won't. Mental illness is like physical illness: The earlier its symptoms are recognized, a doctor called, and proper treatment begun, the better are the chances that the patient will get well again.

It's not just hocus-pocus

Once you consult a reputable doctor, accept his diagnosis and follow his advice. If he tells you the difficulty is mental illness and recommends calling in a psychiatrist, by all means let him do so, just as you would if he recommended a surgeon or a heart specialist or a gynecologist. All these specialists, the psychiatrist with the others, are doctors who have added to their general training in medicine a period of special study in some one phase of the body and its ills.

Do not try to tell the psychiatrist how to treat mental illness any more than you would try to tell a surgeon how to operate. Not long ago an otherwise intelligent and informed man was heard to tell a friend who was worried about her father's state of mind, "Don't get mixed up with psychiatrists; they're fakes; they use a lot of hocus-pocus like hypnotism." Such an attitude is not only ignorant; it is harmful. It reminds one of the days when modern surgery was new. People then were afraid of the new-fangled doctors who "cut a man wide open," and when they could be persuaded to have an operation they preferred to endure the pain of it rather than submit to the "hocus-pocus" of an anesthetic.

Psychiatrists do use hypnotism sometimes, but they use it as a scientific tool in the practice of medicine, not as the entertaining hocus-pocus of the old vaudeville artist or sideshow magician. They use many other methods of treatment too, one of which is the psychoanalysis the general public talks of so glibly but knows so little about.

For many months recently the menu cards of a fashionable restaurant in a midwestern city carried the announcement that patrons could for a fee secure the services of "Madame Sophie, Psychoanalyst." All Sophie did was see the usual handsome, dark man in the same old deck of cards, but she got by for months with her grandiose title because so few people have any notion of what psychoanalysis actually is and does.

Psychoanalysis is a form of treatment for psychiatric disorders that takes many hours over a period of months. It is perfectly respectable and is in no sense a form of entertainment or amusement. It should be used only on the recommendation of a competent psychiatrist, who if he does not practice it himself will suggest a reputable and well-trained psychoanalyst for you to consult.

Advantages of hospital care

If the doctors recommend that your patient be hospitalized for his psychiatric complaint, do not let your old-fashioned ideas of mental hospitals prevent your taking their advice. It is at this point that Sarah is going wrong in her handling of Ted's case. She would not think of taking Ted out of the hospital if he were ill with pneumonia; she would be grateful to have a hospital near by where he could receive the proper care from trained doctors and nurses. But because he needs care in a mental hospital, Sarah is refusing to cooperate with the doctors and is taking matters into her own hands.

Without proper advice and sound information other mothers and wives may also act in this unwise way. Men who develop a psychosis in any one of the armed services are given several weeks or months of treatment by a psychiatrist in a service hospital. In this time some of the men will have recovered sufficiently to be sent home to their families for convalescent care. Of these we shall speak later. Others are still actively ill enough that their doctors consider it necessary to transfer them to another hospital near their home for further treatment. At this point the doctors must have the family's cooperation in making the transfer.

In all too many cases, unfortunately, the family refuse to cooperate and insist that the man be sent home. If they do this because they doubt the diagnosis, because they are sure such a thing couldn't have happened to "our son" or "my husband," they should remember that the doctors' opinion is based on weeks of study and observation, on a lot of facts the family cannot possibly know, and on a long training and experience in mental illness they cannot share.

More often, however, the principal factor in their refusal is the feeling about mental hospitals that we have described, the feeling that is motivating Sarah's action. If you or anyone you know has this mistaken idea, pay a visit to your state mental hospital, or if that is not practicable, read the description of one given in Edith M. Stern's book, *Mental Illness: A Guide for the Family*. You will be surprised to learn about the beauty shops and barbershops, the gardens, the radios, movies, dances, concerts, picnics, and so on that are regular features of any modern mental hospital. It is true that many of our state hospitals and also those maintained by the Veterans Administration are greatly overcrowded and understaffed, but even so they can give better care to those who need it than the family can give at home.

All the loving devotion in the world cannot make the home a satisfactory substitute for the hospital when trained care is needed. Proper equipment for treatment, trained nurses, and the regular routine that is necessary but so difficult to maintain in the average home make the hospital the most desirable place for the mental patient.

Just being there is sometimes an effective treatment in itself, because it gives the patient a chance to catch his emotional breath in impersonal surroundings, away from the strains and entanglements of everyday life. "The best chance of lessening emotional tensions, of slowing down abnormally geared-up minds, is in surroundings created especially for their needs, and not among the demands and competitions of everyday life."

Most important of all the reasons for hospitalization is the doctor's opinion that the patient must be constantly watched, not so often because he is likely to harm others, though he may sometimes do that, but usually because he is dangerous to himself. The person with a psychotic impulse to injure himself or take his own life can be extremely cunning in finding a way to do so. In the home it is impossible to put away every object that he might use for this purpose; in the hospital under the eyes of an experienced staff the danger is much less.

Weigh these factors

There is another side to be considered too. The patient will seldom be the only member of the family. Sarah, for instance, should be thinking not only of Ted, but of Mary and Ruth and Jack. If by taking Ted home, giving up all her time to his care, and sacrificing the other children's social life to his presence in the house, she could make Ted well again, there might be a legitimate reason for her action. But when Ted himself would probably be better off in the hospital, Sarah has no right to sacrifice the whole family's welfare to her concern for him, natural though that concern may be.

This same factor should be considered if there is a choice to be made between a private and a public hospital. If the family can afford the greater privacy and luxury of a private hospital without unduly depriving its healthy members of a comfortable standard of living, all well and good. But if bearing this expense would mean that the other children must forgo any necessities or a good education, the only wise choice is the public hospital. The care it affords will be equal to that of all but the best private institutions and much better than is to be had in many of them. Good private hospitals for mental illness are few and far between, and paying their bills will overtax all but the highest incomes.

In making this decision, the family must remember that the patient may need hospitalization for a period of years. Perhaps he won't, but they should figure on the possibility. If their extra means are limited, they would be wiser to choose the state hospital and save their money to provide extra comforts and pleasures for the patient during his period of convalescence at home.

The law steps in

One unfortunate obstacle to an enlightened attitude regarding hospitalization for mental illness is the antiquated laws that still exist in many of our states. There is no good reason why a competent physician should not be able to secure hospital care for a psychiatric patient as easily as for any other kind. But in this respect our laws and lawyers lag far behind the times. They still, for instance, use the words *insanity* and *lunacy* in these cases, though doctors discarded them years ago. Today *insanity* is only a legal term, not a medical term at all.

Showing more concern for the due process of law than for making adequate care speedily available to the sick, every state but Maryland requires some kind of court commitment for admission to a mental hospital. This is why the military authorities must request the cooperation of the family in transferring a psychotic serviceman to a civilian hospital.

In the more progressive states the necessary commitment is secured by a simple judicial order on the recommendation of two qualified physicians. This procedure is quick and relatively painless for the patient and his family. In other states court proceedings to determine sanity are necessary, but the judges are likely to be more sensible than the laws, to recognize their incompetence in the matter, and to act on medical advice. There are only two states that still force the sick person to go through the ordeal of a sanity trial by jury—a procedure that is about as intelligent as calling in a passer-by on the street to diagnose typhoid fever!

However distasteful the requirements for commitment may be in your state, there is nothing to do but fulfill them for the sake of your relative's health. There is nothing to stop you then from going out and using your influence and your rights as a citizen to get the laws brought up to date.

They do recover

"Once insane always insane" is not true. Psychotics do recover. One half the patients in all mental hospitals leave them recovered or greatly improved, in the majority of cases within eighteen months. In the best institutions the recovery rate is much higher.

It is true that some patients well enough to leave the hospital do have some lingering symptoms, and relapses do occur, but the number who recover give the lie to the old wives' tale that "once you've lost your mind you're never quite right again." In some cases the person is better after his attack than before.

This was true of one young man in whom the effects of a faulty upbringing produced a psychotic breakdown during the last year of his premedical training. He was committed to a mental hospital, and as he began to improve he learned from the doctors what was wrong with his attitudes and habits that produced the breakdown. Applying his intelligence to the remaking of these habits, he came out of the hospital a year later not only well but a stronger personality than before. He went back to school, completed his general training, and then took the special course in surgery. For the past thirteen years he has been an outstandingly successful surgeon in one of our biggest cities.

So do not assume that when you commit your relative to a mental hospital you are "putting him away" for life. Do not abandon him. Write to him frequently and visit him regularly, even though he acts indifferent or hostile to you. That is an expression of his illness. Your constant interest and devotion remain his tie with home and normal living and may be a vital factor in his recovery.

Be careful, however, to observe the rules and regulations of the hospital. They are made for a good reason. For instance, you will probably be asked to limit your gifts to the patient in certain ways and to submit for examination anything you bring him. You may not see the reason for this. You may not see any danger to your relative in the nail file, letter opener, or new tie he wants. And perhaps there is no danger for him. But some depressed patient on the same ward may find your gift and use it to cut the vein in his wrist or hang himself.

Here again it is to your interest to follow the doctors' advice. They will ask your permission before using certain forms of treatment, just as they do in general hospitals before operating. Do not refuse permission just because you have heard "something awful" about the treatment. To save their own reputations, if for no other reason, doctors do not use methods that kill people. Accidental deaths can, of course, occur in any kind of treatment; they do occasionally even in so simple an operation as the removal of the tonsils, yet people go on having their tonsils out to improve their health.

Take the case of Mrs. Morgan, who was asked to permit

the doctors to use shock therapy on her son. This is a form of treatment in which electricity or injections of certain drugs are used to shock the depressed or apathetic patient into the state of awareness he has lost. Mrs. Morgan went to the hospital, talked with the doctors, and signed the permission papers. Then she went in to visit her son William.

At the first sight of his mother, William began begging her to take him home. The doctors and nurses were mean to him, he said; they did "terrible" things to the patients—and he told two or three stories to support his statement. And now they wanted to use this shock treatment on him. It was a horrible thing. It sent patients into convulsions. She must not let them do it to him. She must take him home. Couldn't she see for herself that he was well now?

It would be hard for any mother to resist such a plea. Besides, William sounded perfectly reasonable; he must have got over his trouble. Mrs. Morgan returned to the office, repudiated her permission, and demanded her son's release.

The doctors had a hard time convincing her that William was still very ill. The stories he had told her were entirely without truth, wholly the figments of his sick imagination. At the moment he was lucid and natural, but less than a week before during a depressed period he had tried to commit suicide with his belt buckle. He still had many delusions. He thought the blood in his veins was all water. He had tried not long ago to take the soles off his shoes because they were "phony stuff" he shouldn't have to walk on. A few days before that he had tried to dig the gold crown off one of his teeth because, he said, it wasn't real gold.

These things Mrs. Morgan had not seen in the few minutes she talked with William. Families and friends of psychotic patients must remember that they cannot believe everything the sick man says, no matter how reasonable he sounds. By all means investigate his complaints, ask the hospital authorities about them, but do not act on your relative's say-so. He isn't rational; that's why he's in the hospital.

As for shock therapy, it does give the patient a convulsion;

that is its purpose. The sight is not a pleasant one for the layman, but neither is a surgical operation. And the shock treatment is only one of many the psychiatrist uses, in varying combinations according to the needs of the individual patient.

Do not let your judgment in these matters be swayed by Mrs. Smith down the street who tells you that So-and-so came home from the hospital before the doctor said he could and he got along all right. Perhaps he did; doctors are human and sometimes make mistakes in judgment. But they are certainly better advisers than laymen. They know more psychotic patients than Mrs. Smith does. They know how many times a family has taken a sick relative home against medical advice only to have him get worse, come back to the hospital, and have to start his progress to recovery all over again.

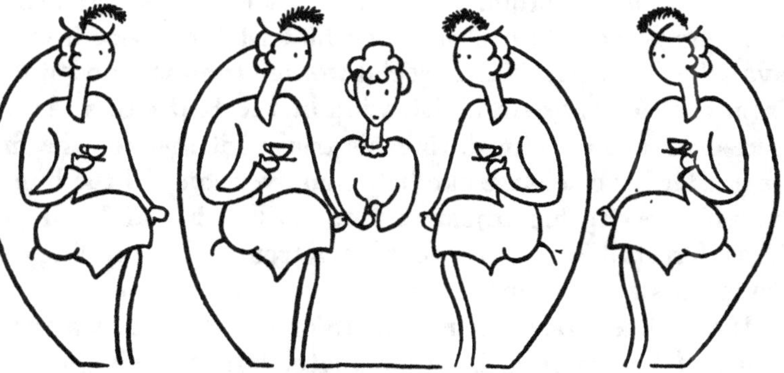

They're no substitute for the doctor

Back home again

When the patient's condition has improved enough for the doctor to consider releasing him from the hospital, he may suggest a trial visit to the family to see how the patient reacts. It is during this trial visit that the family can be most helpful. The doctor will prepare them carefully for the proper handling of the patient, and they should do their best to cooperate, reporting his condition and behavior fairly and accurately to the doctor to help him reach the correct decision about release. Sometimes two or three trial visit periods will be needed before the patient is ready to be discharged.

When he is discharged he will be like the servicemen we spoke of on page 139 — those who have recovered their health sufficiently to be sent home to the family for convalescent care.

Many families with a newly discharged mental patient are like young parents with a new baby in the house; they handle him as if he were the most fragile of glass and are alarmed by every minor symptom. It will ease their minds and benefit the convalescent to call on a psychiatrist for advice if one is available, or a psychiatric social worker from the hospital or from the Veterans Administration or the Red Cross. An experienced eye on him during his trial visit and for the first year after his discharge can help him over some of the bumps he will meet in his adjustment to civilian life and can perhaps forestall a recurrence of his trouble by nipping any symptoms at the start.

If the illness does recur it is unfortunate, just as a recurrence of tuberculosis is unfortunate, but it need mean no more than this. Some patients may be peculiarly susceptible to a recurrence any time they overtax their strength, and some forms of psychosis, such as the manic-depressive, are especially liable to recur. The manic-depressive is often perfectly normal for years between periods of illness, however, and even he may have no more than the first attack.

The hospital doctors will give the family any special advice they may need about caring for their particular convalescent. Perhaps a certain routine will be best for a while, or perhaps there is a particular kind of strain that he must avoid. In the case of servicemen discharged directly from service hospitals to their homes, it will help their families and medical advisers to know something about the nature of the man's breakdown, how it was treated, and what special precautions if any are necessary until he has fully recovered his health. This kind of information can be secured from the military authorities by the family physician or through the Veterans Administration.

Aside from these individual considerations, the family should try to treat their convalescent as nearly as possible like the other members in the family. Don't overdo social life at first, but include him naturally in any regular family activities, such as walking, going to church or the movies, calling on friends, and so on. It may be a good idea to map out his day ahead of time for a while, so the change from the regular routine of the hospital will not be too sudden.

But do not pamper him too much. Because he is probably the oversensitive kind of person who takes the hurts of life too hard, he will always need love and intelligent kindness, but he is no longer the sick man who went away to the hospital. As fast as he is able, he should assume the responsibility for his own life again and get over wanting and expecting the kind of personal service he had in the hospital.

When your man comes home from the hospital, if not before, brace yourself against the unkindness of those who think mental illness is funny or a scandal. There are still so many of these uninformed persons that you are bound to meet some of them. They will look at you pityingly, or, not quite out of your sight and hearing, will tap their foreheads and whisper, "He's crazy." Do not let this upset you unduly. You too probably felt this way once, but now you have learned better.

Don't overprotect your convalescent from these slurs. The sooner he gets used to them and learns to shrug them off as ignorance, the easier and quicker will be his recovery. Act naturally with him and with your friends and neighbors. Neither emphasize his illness nor avoid it. If you try to conceal it, he will feel ashamed and become worried and anxious. This is the surest way to a relapse.

It will be important to keep him pleasantly occupied—with gardening, reading, sports—but he may not be able to go back to work immediately. When he is ready for this, the doctor will advise you of it. He may have to start back on this road gradually too, perhaps working for someone else instead of running his own business at first, or taking a less exacting job for a while. As he gains confidence and strength to meet the normal competition of the workaday world, he will be able to take on more responsibility without danger of undue strain.

The story of Mrs. Gray

In this discussion of the discharged patient we have been assuming that his restoration to full health is possible. In some cases, of course, it may not be. Because of the nature of the illness or the stage it had reached before treatment was begun, only a measure of improvement may be expected. The man may be well enough to be discharged from the hospital and live at home with his family and friends, but he will probably never be able to assume full responsibility for his own life or to go back to work. Then what are you to do, take him home to live with you or leave him in the care of the hospital?

The decision is not one to be made hastily or lightly. You must, as carefully and honestly as you can, weigh what it will mean to him to be at home against the undeniable burden it will put upon the rest of the family to have him there. Be sure, before you bring him home, that you understand what his coming will entail and that you are ready and willing to accept it.

Mrs. Gray had this decision to make. Her husband was a university graduate in pharmacy and a veteran of World War I. Just before the armistice in 1918 he was wounded and had to be in the hospital for some six weeks. During this time he had a mild psychotic breakdown in which he had a delusion about all things green. He was sure, for instance, that the grass around the hospital was a deadly poison which no one must even touch.

He recovered from this quickly and when his wound had healed, he returned to the United States. He and Mrs. Gray were married and went to live in a small town, where he was named manager of a chain drugstore. Anxious to make up for lost time and to get ahead rapidly, Mr. Gray worked very hard and things went well for several years. Then times got bad, the drugstore did not do quite so well, and Mr. Gray began to worry.

One night at a dinner party he leaned across to his wife, pointed at the lime sherbet she was eating, and whispered, "Don't eat that; it's poison." Thinking he was fooling, she just laughed. But a few days later at home he picked the lettuce out of his salad and threw it away, again saying it was poison, and thereafter almost every day he pointed out something green around the house or on the table as being poisonous.

Mrs. Gray was distressed by all this, but she did not realize how ill her husband was until she went over to the drugstore one night to walk home with him. She found him at the prescription counter, "making more money," he said, out of paraffin.

He soon had to give up his job, of course, but for almost a year Mrs. Gray kept him at home with her, hoping that with rest his trouble would clear away. Instead he got worse and worse, until one night he came to her bed and tried to strangle her. Then she knew she could wait no longer; she must put him in a hospital.

She had no trouble getting him admitted to a Veterans Administration hospital, where he stayed for some three years. She went to visit him every week, and he seemed to live for her visits. He trusted her completely and would do anything she told him to. If the nurses had any trouble persuading him to eat or to take his medicine, they just waited until she came, knowing he would do it for her without question.

During this time his condition improved slowly. Finally the doctors told her he was as well as he could ever be. There was no longer any danger of violence, so he could be discharged and live at home with her, but he would always need a great deal of care.

Mrs. Gray had expected this outcome for some time, and her plans were all ready. She had bought a pleasant little house near a lake and set up a gift shop in its front rooms. The back rooms could be made into pleasant quarters for her husband. She knew that having him at home would greatly restrict her activities. She would have to give him a great deal of her time, could never leave him alone, and her social life would be severely limited. But she had no children to consider, and was willing to make the sacrifice herself. So she took Mr. Gray home.

That was eight years ago. They now live a very quiet but companionable life. Mr. Gray talks very little, but he is happy and contented. He reads a lot, mostly in his pharmacy books. Sometimes for short periods he paints or carves plaques to be sold in the gift shop, but he cannot do it for long at a time because the close work makes him nervous. In good weather they go every day to the lake, and sun-bathe or wade in the water along the beach. Twice a week they go to the neighborhood movie, they listen to the radio, and once every week or so they have some friends in for an evening of cards. Mr. Gray does not play or join much in the conversation, but he does not mind having them there.

Despite the decidedly limited scope of her life, Mrs. Gray is not unhappy. She knew what it would mean to her when she took her husband from the hospital. With the money she receives each month from the government as her husband's pension plus the income from her gift shop, she is able to manage reasonably well financially. And she finds the satisfactions denied her in her home life in the development of her now established and flourishing little business.

Some do's and don'ts

Let the doctor be your guide. No layman can find the way, for himself or for another, through the jungles of severe mental illness. The guidance of a good doctor is as necessary here as in any other kind of illness. Doctors are not infallible, but they have special training and experience, which is certainly more reliable than the positive but uninformed opinions of the neighbor across or down the street.

You must cooperate with the doctor in providing him or the psychiatric social workers who assist him with honest, accurate information about his patient. You would not expect him to make an accurate diagnosis and give you proper treatment if you falsified your physical symptoms. Neither can he do so if, out of false pride or shamed reluctance, you conceal or gloss over the truth about psychiatric symptoms. And in most cases you of the family must provide this information; the patient himself will be too confused and irrational to do so.

If the doctor advises hospitalization, arrange for it, whatever is required, and let his be the sole decision about the time for release from the hospital. When he says the patient is ready to go home, you may act on his opinion without fear of consequences. If he tells you to watch for certain signs of possible recurrence, do so carefully but without fear. Fear is contagious and your convalescent will sense your feeling it, his confidence will be shaken by it, and his recovery will be retarded.

Don't be frightened by mere words. It has been said that words alone can kill people, by the worry they cause. Through associations over long years, words like *insane, crazy, asylum, psychiatrist,* and *commitment* have acquired the power to arouse in us powerful emotions that have little relation to their actual meaning. Do not let these emotions dictate your actions or direct your thinking. Try always to look behind the words for the actual facts.

Here is an example of the injustice "words" can cause.

Carl suffered a breakdown while he was in training. His illness was diagnosed as a manic-depressive psychosis, and after six months of treatment in an army hospital he was transferred to a veterans' hospital for mental patients. At the end of four months there, he was entirely recovered. Released, he applied for a job in a large manufacturing concern, telling them frankly about his illness. The personnel officer investigated his record and gave him a job as a machine operator. He proved a valuable employee and he was happy in his work.

Harry lived in the same town. His service was in the navy, and his breakdown occurred after his ship was torpedoed. He too was diagnosed as manic-depressive. After several months in a navy hospital he was to be transferred to a veterans' hospital, but his family objected strenuously and had him sent home instead. There he got so much worse that they had to put him in a hospital. No beds were then available in the veterans' hospital, so they had him committed to the state hospital for mental illness. Here he too recovered quickly and was discharged.

Harry applied for a job at the same place Carl was working, and he told the interviewer his story. But this time, after investigating his record, the personnel officer refused him a job on the grounds that he was unemployable.

Discouraged, Harry took his problem to the service officer of one of the veterans' organizations, who happened to know Carl's story. The service officer went to the company's office and asked why they had made such different decisions in these two cases that were so much alike. "But they aren't alike," said the personnel officer. "Harry was committed to a state hospital; Carl never was."

"What difference does that make?" asked the service officer.

"Well, if a man is committed to a state hospital it must mean he's insane. So obviously we don't want him; he's not employable."

Knowing that this is not true, the service officer insisted that the personnel man go with him to the government psychiatrist and get his ideas straight. Harry and Carl suffered from the same type of illness, said the psychiatrist; both had recovered, and one was as employable as the other. Their cases were just handled differently because of circumstances. Harry's commitment made no difference whatever.

When the personnel officer understood the facts instead

of reacting emotionally to the word *commitment*, he hired Harry and found him just as good a worker as Carl.

Don't blame your serviceman for his breakdown. Inability to endure the conditions of military service is his misfortune perhaps, but not his fault.

Remember too that you are dealing with someone who is sick, not wicked, weak-willed, or simply perverse. Focus your emotions on this fact instead of being exasperated by his unreasonable behavior and trying to account for it. His stubbornness, his abuse of you, his lack of cleanliness, his queer ideas — all these are symptoms of his illness. They are to be taken no more personally, with no more anguish or distress, than is vomiting with a stomach disorder.

Don't try to argue with a psychotic patient. You can't make him see reason; you will only excite him. His mind is not working the way it did or the way yours does, and he is not aware of this fact. This too is part of his illness; doctors call it "lack of insight." Be patient with him, but firm if necessary. You must make the decisions and carry them out.

Don't lie to him. If he must go to the hospital, for instance, tell him honestly but quietly where he is going. Don't, just to make things easier for yourself, tell him you are taking him for an automobile ride or on a picnic. His mind is not so confused that he won't know the difference when he arrives. Keep his confidence in you and what you say; it will stand you in good stead later.

Don't make up foolish stories for your friends and neighbors. When it becomes necessary, tell them frankly what is wrong with your relative and where he has gone for treatment. If you lie it will be found out, and your attempt at concealment will only add fuel to the fire of gossip. Be straightforward about the whole matter; you have nothing to be ashamed of, whatever others may think, and your own acceptance of the misfortune will of itself force them to take the same attitude. Remember that anyone who today thinks that mental illness is either funny or shameful is ignorant, and at least a hundred years behind the times.

Don't sacrifice four or five lives in a vain attempt to salvage one. That is, don't surrender the interests of the entire family, financially or socially, to an oversentimental regard for the one sick member. The chances are you will not help him in the least by doing so.

Adolescents especially have not the wisdom or the experience necessary to withstand social pressure. If your children's young friends make fun of their brother, mimic his oddities, say unkind things about him, or are afraid of him, your children will themselves be psychologically injured. They will feel a vague personal shame, will become overly defensive, will avoid bringing their friends home, perhaps withdraw from outside friendships altogether. Many a developing personality has been seriously warped by community reactions to a mentally deranged relative kept at home. You have no right to subject your children to this risk if it can be avoided.

Don't go looking for psychiatric symptoms in yourself and your friends; you will find them. We all have quirks and eccentricities, but that does not mean that we are all mentally ill. It is only when a person's behavior becomes seriously different from what it has been that one need suspect mental illness and call the doctor.

This is especially applicable within the family when one of its members has had a breakdown. That one of you has got sick does not mean that it is only a matter of time till the rest of you come down with the same complaint. Psychosis is not a contagious disease, nor is any inherited tendency toward it so strong as that. Doctors are inclined to believe that the tendency to certain kidney ailments runs in families, but if one member of your family had to go to the hospital for diabetes you would not go into a panic every time one of the others reached for a lump of sugar.

Be sensible about this, and you will save yourself a lot of needless and foolish anxiety.

Keep a firm check on your own behavior, your own self-control. Don't fuss and fret, wring your hands, weep, and otherwise behave so hysterically that the doctor must calm you down before he can take care of your son or husband. There will be many things for you to attend to, and you cannot handle them efficiently if you lose your head. Besides, nervous fussiness or anxiety will have the worst possible effect on the sick person. Confused and excited himself, he needs calm, not turmoil, around him.

And finally, the overanxious, oversolicitous relative is a nuisance to the doctors and the nurses. One distraught mother whose son had suddenly to be put in a hospital actually wrote ten letters in one day to the hospital superintendent. And when she came to visit her son, she walked on tiptoe,

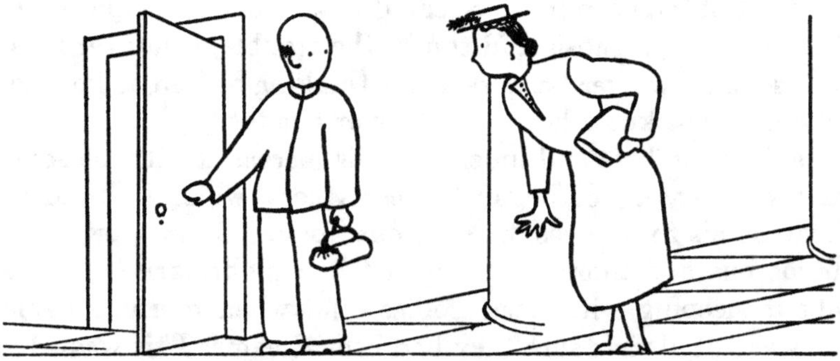

Don't act worse than the patient you're visiting!

shushed everybody in sight, peered nervously around the door before entering the room, and in the office suggested, cautioned, and questioned until the doctor began to wonder whether it wasn't she who should be in the hospital instead of her son.

Be kind and understanding, but do not pamper him. You do not want him to remain an invalid, and the mind as well as the body grows stronger with reasonable exercise. Don't wait on him hand and foot; don't make all his decisions for him. Give him a chance to become his own boss again. But do not force him toward this goal faster than he is able to go; failures will weaken the self-confidence he and you are striving to strengthen.

Do all you can to improve the lot of all mental patients. Work to erase in your neighborhood, your city, and your state the undeserved social stigma that makes mental illness so much harder for the patient and his family. Give your active support to any proposed legislation for the improvement of state hospitals, the creation of municipal or county mental hygiene clinics, and the modernizing of state sanity laws. Use what your own experience has taught you to help make the same misfortune easier for others.

Sarah's tomorrow

Sarah, then, may be making a serious mistake in taking Ted out of the hospital to be cared for at home. She questions the doctors' diagnosis and thinks the trouble, whatever it is, will soon blow over because she is thinking of Ted as he was. She does not know how his behavior changed.

As his conflicts and inner tensions increased without solution or release, Ted began to hear voices, which he tried to answer; his fixed ideas, like the one about yellow, grew more numerous and more annoying; he had nightmarish dreams about sleeping with dead bodies, and when morning came he was not always sure they had been dreams. This was why the doctors called his trouble a psychosis and put him in the hospital for his own protection. His condition has improved, but he is still far from well.

It is impossible to predict what will happen to him at home. There is of course a chance that he will continue to get better, but it is far more likely that he will remain the same or get worse again. When this happens Sarah will realize that she cannot take proper care of him, that his symptoms will not just clear away, that she cannot keep the truth from the neighbors. And if she is honest she will soon have to admit that by letting Ted, in his disordered mental state, make a spectacle of himself in front of visitors or on the street, she is giving thoughtless people far more cause to talk about him than if he were in the state hospital.

When she realizes that she must send Ted to a hospital,

she may take her problem to her family doctor, to the Red Cross or one of the veterans' service organizations, or to the Veterans Administration. If a bed is available in the nearest veterans' hospital, Ted will be admitted there; if not, arrangements will be made for his care at the state mental hospital. In neither case will Sarah have any fees or expenses to pay.

Whether Ted eventually recovers or improves enough to return home will depend on the nature of his illness and the way it responds to the doctors' handling of it. In any case, his progress has almost certainly been retarded by the interruption of the treatment.

Sarah can hardly be blamed if she feels bitter about what has happened, if she says "The war did this to Ted." But did it? There seems little doubt that the demands of military service precipitated Ted's breakdown, but whether or not they caused it is a debatable question. On the answer to it will depend the pension and benefits to which Ted is entitled. If the rating board decides that his illness is service-connected, that is, was incurred in the line of military duty, his disability will be rated total and permanent, and he will, for the duration of his illness, receive the same pension and benefits awarded Joe for his paralysis. Ted, however, is in one way much more fortunate than Joe. There is a better chance of Ted's return to full and normal health.

If he is mentally hurt . . .
GIVE HIM A CHANCE

Edith and Sam

Standing quietly beside the tracks, Edith, the fifth of the waiting women, appears quite the opposite of Sarah. She is a young woman in her late twenties, the mother of three-year-old twins. Smart in her black suit with touches of white, she looks calm and poised, but her mind too is in turmoil, a whirlpool of uncertainty and questions.

Edith is waiting for her husband Sam, who after two years of army service, is returning from overseas with an N-P discharge for psychoneurosis.

What does it mean? Edith wonders. What is wrong with Sam? His letter telling her he was coming home sounded so depressed that Edith could not imagine what had happened to him. She couldn't believe he had "gone to pieces," as he put it. Not when he had been getting along so well.

Sam had always got along well. In high school and college he never had to say "I don't know." How she and the others in his classes envied him! They said, half exasperated, that they believed he could recite his lessons backward. When she came to know him better, she found it hard to believe that he got so scared before examinations that he'd vomit, and would sweat till his shirt was wet. It certainly didn't slow up his thinking any; he always topped the class.

Sam had never got over that queer scaredness. It was something like stage fright, only worse—though Edith could remember stories of great pianists who were so paralyzed by fear before every performance that their managers had literally to push them out onto the platform. She had watched Sam go through this agony a few times after they were married, when there was something special coming up in which he wanted to do exceptionally well. It was difficult for him to describe the sick feeling he had at such times. It was as though something terrible were going to happen, he told her, though he could never name any one thing he feared.

Surely it hadn't bothered him much in the army. He had started in as a private and risen to first lieutenant in two years. He'd been so pleased when he was chosen for officers' training; it had been worrying him that he wasn't providing better for her and the children.

And now this! It couldn't mean that Sam was losing his mind. His letters sounded the same as ever, only so utterly discouraged. And apologetic somehow, as though he'd done something to be ashamed of. But she knew Sam better than to believe that.

What will this mean for their future? Will Sam be able to work again? Will he be able to study medicine if they can manage the time and money? Edith knows that Sam has never given up his hope of being a doctor, even though their marriage and the twins' coming so soon have forced him to be content with his B.S. and a laboratory job for a while. She suspects his parents have been planning to give him the chance to realize his dream when the war is over.

Sam's parents. How will they take this discharge? His university professor father and his novelist mother, both so brilliant themselves, so proud of Sam, and so ambitious for his success. Will they be upset? Perhaps not. Perhaps they'll understand this thing that has hit Sam, since his father has suffered for years from nervous indigestion.

What does it mean?

Edith's bewildered questions are those of most laymen confronted with a diagnosis of psychoneurosis, and of many servicemen too. Not long ago one of these men wrote to an advice-to-the-lovelorn columnist: "I've been discharged for psychoneurosis. What does it mean? Do they think I'm crazy? I don't feel any different than I did before."

Psychoneurosis has become something of a diagnostic scrap basket. Like *shell shock* in World War I, the term is so loosely used that it can mean anything from an abnormal fear of dogs to a panicky fear of crowds so overwhelming that the victim cannot stir outside his own doorway. Military authorities are confronted with something that makes a man unfit for service. It is not a physical disability; it is not a psychosis. So it goes into the great undifferentiated class of psychoneurosis.

The label certainly does not mean that the man is insane; he may not even be noticeably queer in any way. It does not mean he is a coward, or that he has not tried his best to fit into the service. It does not mean that he has inherited some taint of character or will transmit one to his children by inheritance. It does not mean he is lacking in intelligence.

Psychoneurotics (or neurotics; the two are the same) are more likely to be above average in intelligence. They may be high-strung, nervous people, oversensitive, overconscientious, ambitious, with a strong sense of responsibility and devotion to duty. Or they may be such warmhearted, generous individuals, so closely attached to family, friends, and home that all their acts and judgments are colored by their feelings. They may be exceedingly well behaved, never troublesome, precise in their ways, always wanting things in place and living always according to a careful schedule.

But whatever their personalities, they are all individuals who cannot face certain kinds or degrees of difficulty without experiencing mental and physical symptoms that handicap them in some degree for the daily business of living.

The troublesome symptoms may be legion. Among the commonest are profound exhaustion, anxiety, depression, feelings of guilt, formless fears, panic, chronic indecision, worry, sleeplessness, and the many physical symptoms that emotion can produce, such as weakness, headaches, stomach pain, dizzy spells, diarrhea, sweating, uncontrollable trembling, palpitation of the heart, and vomiting. Less often there may be blindness, deafness, inability to speak, or paralysis of some part of the body.

Most of these symptoms may occur in a perfectly normal

person, of course. The difference is that the psychoneurotic suffers them more intensely and with less external cause. For example: To be afraid if a gangster pokes a gun in your ribs some dark night on a lonely street is perfectly normal. To be afraid when you are sitting comfortably at home in a brightly lighted room with friends is not so normal. To be anxious about a loved one who is seriously ill is normal. To feel the same sense of impending disaster without any cause one can name is not so normal.

The name doesn't matter

The psychoneurotic is not a freak; he belongs to a goodly company. It includes not only 90 per cent of all those given N-P discharges from the army, but thousands and thousands of civilians as well. All of us know people who are badly adjusted to life, can't get along with people, live in constant fear of failure, turn every molehill into a mountain. It is

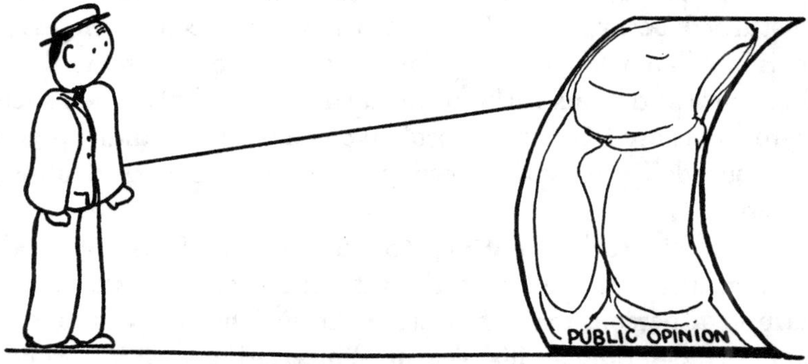

The mirror exaggerates!

estimated that one half the persons who seek advice from doctors do so for complaints that are psychological in origin. Some experts would put the proportion much higher, and one has gone so far as to say, "If you're not neurotic, you're not normal."

That is an exaggeration of course, but its point is true; there are a great many neurotics among us.

Psychoneurosis occurs in all degrees, from mild to severe. Doctors disagree about where to draw the line between "neurotic behavior" in the normal person and psychoneurosis as a mental illness. Some say that anyone who is *excessively* shy or aggressive or moody or timid or suspicious or excitable is neurotic. They would include the banker with a twitching tic in his eyelid, the schoolboy who stammers, the maiden aunt who has constant headaches, the business executive who watches the clock to make sure his employees come and go on time. Others call this use of the word ridiculous, preferring to keep it for symptoms that are more nearly incapacitating.

For the layman this argument over a name is of no matter. The important thing is not what you call it, but what it does to you. If you have a slight head cold, you don't worry because the doctor might call it a respiratory disease. Only if it is bad enough to keep you in bed and home from work do you consider it an illness. In the same way, you need not be disturbed because you have an occasional sleepless night, a period of anxiety or depression now and then, or some fleeting aches and pains without physical disease. Only when such symptoms are frequent or prolonged enough to handicap you in your daily activities need you become concerned about them.

Psychoneurosis is nothing to laugh about. It is not fatal, but neither is a broken ankle. Like the broken ankle, it can cripple a person, make him limp through life in pain or discomfort, clouding all his pleasures, interfering with his friendships, and lowering his effectiveness at work and in the general art of living. The psychoneurotic is not a happy person.

Yet from the viewpoint of society, psychoneurosis may be a good thing. Many of the world's most brilliant men of science, literature, and art have been driven to their accomplishments by the inner pressure of a neurosis. To overcome their mental and emotional handicaps in one direction, they develop greater abilities, push farther and harder, in another. It is for this reason that psychiatrists occasionally refuse to interfere; they see that "To cure a neurosis might spoil a poet" or a musician or a sculptor.

Gauguin, whose paintings give many of us deep pleasure, almost certainly would not have done those paintings except for what we now call a psychoneurosis. America's beloved Abraham Lincoln was psychoneurotic, and so in lesser degrees were Charles Lamb, Charles Darwin, Samuel Johnson, and many more of history's great men.

Some outward signs

Not all the symptoms we have listed are present in every case. From those that are present the psychiatrist decides whether the psychoneurosis is anxiety type, hysteria, neurasthenia, or psychasthenia.

The anxiety type is commonest among servicemen. It is characterized by a constant condition of morbid fear and anxiety, and its principal symptoms are nervous irritability, anxious dread of the future for no namable reason, sweating, vomiting, diarrhea, trembling, and feelings of suffocation.

Hysteria as a type of psychoneurosis is not the hysteria of the screaming woman. It is a loss or disturbance of function in some part of the body. The patient may lose his memory, be insensible to pain when cut or pricked with a pin, or be paralyzed in his arm, hand, leg, or foot. There is nothing physically wrong with the body in these cases; the trouble is entirely functional. The patient *could* move his arm, for instance, but he *can't.*

In neurasthenia the main symptoms are a profound fatigue and aches and pains so numerous that the patient's account of them is said to be an "organ recital." Neurasthenia is not common among servicemen, nor is psychasthenia, the kind of neurosis in which the patient suffers from a kind of mental paralysis that makes the simplest decision extraordinarily difficult. It may take him many minutes to decide whether to wear the green or the blue tie, whether to have his breakfast eggs boiled or scrambled. He is also likely to suffer from an urge to perform some simple act over and over again, perhaps to wash his hands every few minutes, to count the cracks in the sidewalk as he walks to work, or to touch every tree or post he passes. He knows this is absurd but he cannot control the impulse.

How will he be?

We have given these brief descriptions of the kinds of psychoneurosis only to take the mystery out of their names if you should encounter them. You need not concern yourself about them; it is the doctor's province to make the diagnosis. What the families and friends of psychoneurotic servicemen want to know is what their men will be like when they come home.

In many cases they will not be very different from what they were when they went away. They will be so little changed that even close friends may wonder (silently we hope!) why they are not still in uniform. The reason is that their difficulty is of a kind that does not bother them in civilian life; it handicaps them only in military service.

Take the case of Tom. A sensitive and gentle man, a devoted husband, and a kind father, Tom was also a very good lawyer. But he did not make a good soldier. For one thing he was incurably clumsy in using his hands, but the chief reason was that he was gun-shy; he would jump every time he heard a shot, and his hands would tremble so that he could not hold a rifle.

His buddies teased him a great deal about this, but Tom had a lot of common sense and he was good-natured. He would just retort, "Well, I'd like to see what you'd do with a lawbook or before a jury." Tom was sorry he couldn't meet the army requirements, but he did not let his failure in this make him think he could not do anything else either. He tried to overcome the difficulty, but no matter how hard he tried, whenever a gun went off near him he would jump and tremble in spite of himself.

Obviously, Tom was of little use to the army; so he was given an N-P discharge. But back in civilian life again, where he doesn't have to hear or handle guns, he is just as intelligent, gentle, kind, and successful as before.

Some discharged psychoneurotics will actually be better than they were before. Their personalities will be stronger because their army experience and the doctor's interpretation of it will have made them understand themselves better. This is the case with Larry. For twelve years Larry had been unhappy in his job. He did well enough at it, but he didn't like it. Working over long rows of figures in an office all alone, he would sometimes go a whole day or more without seeing anyone.

When Larry went into the army, he got upset during the rifle practice in basic training because he was told to focus each shot on an imaginary Jap or German. He lost sleep over this, ate poorly, and became so unable to function that he had to be discharged. During his illness the army psychiatrist explained to him that he had an unusual degree of sensitivity to people. He was warm and generous, fond of people in general, and interested in their problems. That's why the rifle practice upset him so; it went against something very deep and fine inside him. And that was why he was unhappy in his lonely job back home; he needed some kind of work that would bring him into close contact with people, lots of them and of all kinds.

Larry went home, not to return to his old job, but to take up the study of social work at the state university. He is getting along well and will undoubtedly be successful. He is already happier than he has been for years, and he would be quite all right if it were not for one thing: he has a piece of paper with the word *psychoneurosis* on it. He understands what it means, but the people around him do not. They raise their eyebrows because he is not in uniform, and when he tries to explain, they don't quite understand.

When the man comes home with some of his symptoms unrelieved by treatment, what may you expect? You may notice the change first when he tries to pick up a glass or light a cigarette; his hand trembles and he can't stop it. Then you may notice that he can't control his emotions. When some distressing subject is being discussed, or when he has had a tiring experience, he may leave the room abruptly or even break into tears.

He may be irritable and restless, unable to sleep, prowling the house at night while the rest of you are in bed. Or if he does sleep, he may suffer from combat dreams, in which he goes through again the awful sights and sounds and smells of the battlefield. He may dream he is once more in the falling plane, that bombs are dropping all around him, that he is surrounded by a ring of bayonets.

He may be oversensitive to noise, jumping out of his chair and trembling at the slam of a door or the ringing of the telephone. He loves his children, but the sound of their feet on the cement walk outside the window, the noise of their laughter and their roller skates may make him so nervous and tense that he wants to scream. In trying not to give way to this, he may get cross and unduly severe.

Or he may be simply exhausted, tired out in a way that you and I have never been tired. Even the smallest effort for us may be too much for him. He decides to fix the light in the hallway, but by the time he has his tools assembled he's weak and shaky, his heart pounding, his forehead wet with perspiration. He doesn't know what is wrong, but he has to go and lie down.

Even the little things of life may be too much for him; they may seem so many that he just can't start doing any of them. Many a psychoneurotic would recognize the state of mind described in this little verse:

> There was an old man my grandfather knew
> Who had so many things he wanted to do,
> Whenever he thought it was time to begin
> He couldn't because of the state he was in.

Or your serviceman may have one or more of the physical symptoms we have described. This is the hardest part of psychoneurosis for the layman to understand, and it is often a source of bewilderment, even resentment, for the man himself. He has this pain in his stomach, for instance, but the doctor tells him there is nothing wrong with his stomach. How is he to believe that? He knows he has the pain. And his civilian friends shake their heads: "Uh-huh. Just imagination. He's a slacker, faking this pain to get out of fighting." Well, he isn't.

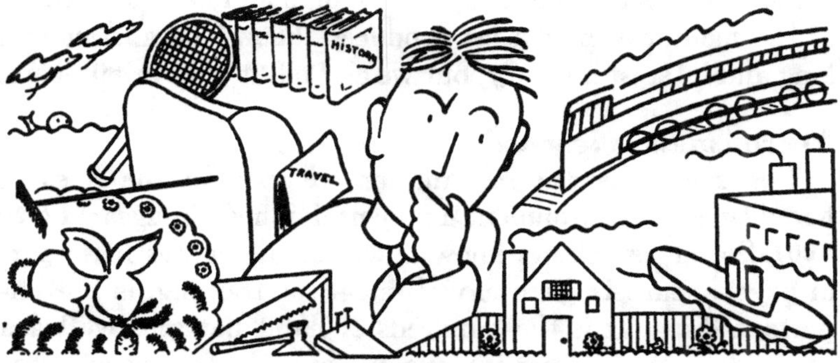

He can't begin, the state he's in

There are, of course, malingerers, fakers, and goldbrickers in the army as well as in civilian life—men who have no symptoms, who make them up or lie about them, knowing all the while that they are doing so But the psychoneurotic really has the aches and pains he describes. It is true that they are not caused by any injury or disease of the body organs; they result from improper functioning.

Suppose you overeat and your stomach gets upset; you may have a headache as well as distress in your stomach; yet nothing is organically wrong in your head. In a somewhat similar way, the emotional upsets that constitute psychoneurosis may upset the functioning of the body so that physical pain or distress results.

Thousands of civilians who go to doctors with what they think is physical sickness are suffering from these psychoneurotic troubles. Yet doctors find it the hardest thing in the world to convince them of this truth. Even if the patient understands that mental turmoil can bring on physical disease, he is sure this is not the case with him, because he is unaware of any problem serious enough to cause his pain.

This is equally true of the fears and anxieties for which the patient can name no cause, the weakness and tiredness that is not explained by physical fatigue, and the paralysis or blindness or deafness that have no basis in damage to the eyes, the ears, or the paralyzed parts.

How can such things happen to a man and he not be aware of the mental conflict that produces them. The answer is a long and interesting story, but we can tell it only briefly here.

Nervousness is learned

You remember the explanation we gave of the roles of heredity and environment in mental illness (pages 117 to 120). So far as doctors know now, heredity plays little part in psychoneurosis; here environment, or training, is the important thing. It is the hundreds of habit patterns we learn as children that determine our susceptibility to neurosis as adults.

Pavlov, the Russian scientist, began to make this fact clear to us. Knowing that a dog's mouth will water at the sight of food, Pavlov tried the experiment of ringing a bell each time the dog was given food. When he had done this long enough for the dog to associate the sound of the bell with the coming of food, Pavlov tested his response to the bell alone. Sure enough, the dog's mouth watered and his tail wagged in happy excitement, just as they had at the sight of food. The instinctive physical reaction to food had been transferred to the associated sound of the bell.

To this process and its result the psychologists gave the names *conditioning* and *conditioned reflex*. We can call them simply *learning* and a *learned response*.

This same process goes on in human beings. A baby will cry when it is allowed to fall, not from pain at hitting the floor — it isn't dropped that far — but from instinctive fright at the sensation of falling. If a bell is rung each time the baby drops, it will soon cry at the sound of the bell when lying safely in its crib, not falling at all. This reaction to the bell is a learned response, just like the dog's response to the bell.

Suppose a child four or five years old, whom we'll call Ned, is sitting on a window sill watching a parade. Some nervous adult notices him, grabs at him, and in fright says, "Don't ever do that again. You might fall and kill yourself." A month or so later Ned is on a boat. He's standing at the railing enjoying the wind and the water. Again he is snatched out of harm's way with the terrifying admonition against falling. A year later he is clambering up the scaffolding of a new house near home. The little friend who is with him loses his footing, falls, and is killed or badly injured. Again the child, frightened enough already by the incident, is nervously and solemnly warned about the danger of falling.

The chances are great that when Ned grows up he will still experience all the sensations of panic every time he finds himself in a high place. Through the same process of conditioning that made the baby feel fright at the sound of a bell, Ned will react to heights with a fear of falling.

In the story of Tom the lawyer on page 164, his jumping and trembling at the sound or sight of a gun is almost certainly the same kind of learned response as the baby's fear of a bell and Ned's fear of heights. Tom has forgotten the experiences that made him gun-shy, but their effects are still active in his life. Why has he forgotten them, if they made such a lasting impression on him? Because they have been pushed out of his memory into the reservoir of experience that is called the subconscious mind.

Let us think of each person's mind as working on three levels of awareness. The first of these we call the conscious mind, and in it lie the things the person is seeing, feeling, or thinking about at the present moment. On the second level lie the things he knows but isn't thinking about. He knows the name of his father, for instance, but isn't thinking of it at the moment; he can, however, instantly recall it to his conscious mind if he wants to. This second level of things remembered may be called the pro-conscious or fore-conscious.

When experiences or thoughts or feelings are very unpleasant, the conscious mind wants to be rid of them so as to be at peace again. So it pushes or represses them into the third level, which is called the subconscious. Between the first two levels and the third there appears to be some sort of barrier, because the experience that has passed into the subconscious cannot easily be recalled. To reverse the familiar phrase, it is forgotten but not gone. We are no longer conscious or aware of it, but it is active in our lives.

These painful experiences that, along with all their mental and emotional associations, are buried deep in the subconscious form what are called complexes. They are like sore spots you don't know you have, but when anything rubs them or presses against them, they make their presence felt by pain and distress. Young Ned's fear of falling, Tom's early experiences with guns, have become such complexes. A high place or the sight of a gun presses on the buried sore, and it responds by making Ned get weak and dizzy and Tom jump and tremble.

The melody lingers on

A good example of this subconscious influence is reported by Dr. David H. Fink in his book, *Release from Nervous Tension.* He once had a patient who suffered from an extremely severe case of asthma. He had a bad spell of coughing and choking every time he got within sight or smell of roses. After a period of examination and treatment, Dr. Fink decided his patient's trouble came from some mental association with roses rather than from any physical allergy to them. So he put the matter to the test. The next time his patient came to the office he saw on the table a beautiful bouquet of roses. They brought on a very bad attack of his asthma, and he was naturally indignant that Dr. Fink should have had roses around when he was expected. His indignation gave way to consternation when Dr. Fink showed him that the "roses" were made of paper.

Was he imagining these attacks of asthma? Was he just

faking them? Of course not. He and the doctor both knew they were much too severe for that. He was reacting to roses exactly as Tom does to a gun or Ned to a high place.

Dr. Fink immediately set out to unbury the complex that was causing this reaction to roses, even to paper ones. It took a long time, but the memories finally came back. As a young man, the patient had been very much in love with a girl whom he thought of as incorruptibly good and pure, and he tried to express his feeling by sending her each day a few roses.

For a time all went well, but he was too poor to marry her right away, and before he was ready she broke her engagement and married another man. For a long time the patient felt very bad about the whole affair; then he decided it must not spoil his life, that he had better go on about the business of making a living and finding another girl. He did so very successfully. His love for the first girl, his wounded vanity, and his shattered ideals faded so completely from his conscious mind that he forgot all about the incident. But it did not disappear from his life; it had simply passed into his subconscious mind, to make its presence felt by an increasingly severe reaction every time he saw the roses he had once associated with the girl he loved.

Laura's trouble was of exactly the same nature. She and her mother were very close to each other, and when her mother died, Laura was inconsolable for a long time. She felt utterly lost, was nervous, couldn't sleep or eat. Every time she thought of her mother, which she did often as she went lovingly through her clothes and personal belongings, she got faint, cried, and felt an uneasy heaviness in her stomach.

After a while she began to get over this unnatural grief. Her friends persuaded her to leave the old house, get herself a job, go out more often for good times with them. Gradually Laura's thoughts of her mother faded to a pleasant memory and she was quite happy again.

Except for one thing. She was sure she was not well. So often she had a queer feeling of faintness, of wanting to cry, of an uncomfortable lump in her stomach. These spells came on her without warning or reason; she might be looking in a shop window on her way to work, or be listening to the music at dinner in some restaurant. She could not imagine what was causing these attacks.

Fortunately her doctor could tell her, once he had made sure there was no physical cause for them. All her intense emotion over the death of her mother was still active in her subconscious mind, and whenever she saw something, perhaps a hat in a shop window, or heard something, perhaps a song in a restaurant, that reminded her of her mother, this emotion came to life in the physical symptoms she had once experienced in connection with her mother's death. She was quite unaware of this process, but it was taking place just the same.

Even dogs break down

To understand this process a little better, we must go back to Pavlov's experiments with dogs. Having learned that dogs could be conditioned to respond to a bell with all the signs of hunger, Pavlov wondered whether they could also be taught to show fear without cause, and if so, what would happen if the two responses were brought into conflict. To find out, he taught a dog to associate anticipation of food with a low-toned bell; then this same dog was given a light electric shock each time he heard a high-toned bell. The dog soon transferred to the sound of the second bell all the fear reactions aroused by the shock; the high-pitched sound alone would make him cower in a corner, his tail between his legs, his ears down, his mouth dry.

When the two responses had been thoroughly established, the bells were gradually changed. The low-toned bell that meant food was slowly raised in pitch; the high-toned bell that meant shock was slowly lowered, a little each day. For a time the dog didn't notice the difference, but as the two bells approached the same pitch, he began to show confusion and bewilderment. He couldn't tell the difference between them.

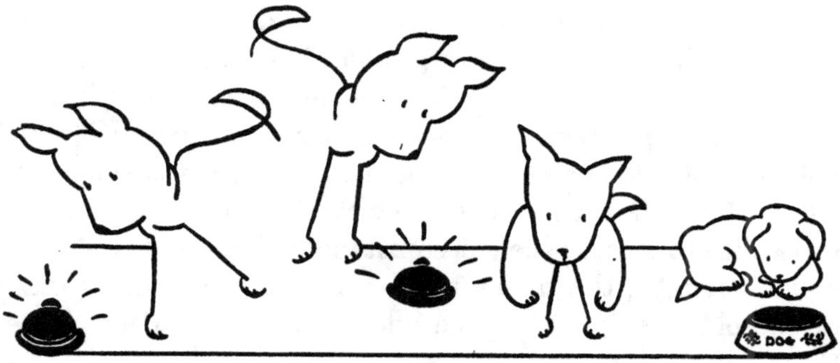

It can happen to dogs

He didn't know whether to expect food or to be afraid, so he crept into a corner, trembled all over, refused to eat or drink, and snapped irritably at everyone who came near him. At times he would slobber; at other times his mouth would be bone dry. Sometimes his heart would pound wildly. He had developed a neurosis.

People laugh at the idea of a dog's having a nervous breakdown, but it can happen and it does. Neuroses have been produced in cats, pigs, and sheep as well as in dogs, by this same process of bringing two learned responses or habit patterns into conflict.

Pioneer hunters on the western prairies often saw this same thing happen in whole herds of buffalo. And they made practical use of it. Picking a small herd, one of the hunting party would shoot into it. The herd would stop, then by instinct whirl about and move as one in another direction. Another hunter would fire at the ground in front of them and again they would stop, wheel, and change direction. This was continued until the bewildered animals, paralyzed by the conflict between their instinct to turn and their fear of the shot that came whenever they did turn, stood helpless and terrified, to be shot down one by one to the last animal.

Pulled two ways

The symptoms of the soldier who breaks down in combat are no more imagined, no more faked, no more the sign of weakness, than were those of Pavlov's dog or those of the prairie buffalo. For they are produced by the same process. In combat men are faced with the fundamental conflict between their instinct for self-preservation and their learned obligation to do their duty. The instinct impels them to run when life itself is threatened; society has taught them it is cowardice to do so. When circumstances give these two forces equal strength, the man's mind becomes the meeting place of the old unstoppable force and immovable object. Something has to give way.

The story of Corporal Jones illustrates this clearly. Jones was picked to lead a patrol across a field that was under heavy artillery fire. Having been in the line for twenty-eight days, Jones was physically worn out; he'd already had enough artillery fire to last him a lifetime, and remembering the close calls he'd had he was thoroughly scared.

There were two things he could do: He could go through the fire scared as he was, in which case he'd be a brave guy; or he could refuse to go — and be dubbed a coward. He wasn't a coward and a coward was the last thing he wanted to be called. So a war began in Jones's mind — his conscience on one side and his instinct for self-preservation on the other. "What the devil, if I go out there I'll get blown to hell; if I don't go out there I'll be yellow and the whole outfit will know it."

Jones's mind had gone through this before, but never for very long; his conscience had never had much trouble winning out. But this time fatigue was fighting on the side of the instinct to run away. Jones couldn't decide what to do, and the tug of war in his mind got worse and worse.

Jones's tired conscious mind could not find a way out of the impasse, but his subconscious mind could. Something stronger than his will power took over the deciding. Suddenly his hands began to shake violently. He didn't understand what was wrong and tried to control them, but the harder he tried the harder they shook. His problem was solved. He could not hold his rifle, so he could not lead the patrol.

You can't know the half of it

The civilian must remember that he can never fully appreciate the emotional experience that men like Corporal Jones have gone through. Father, mother, wife, and friend may see motion pictures of combat, may read the war stories in magazines and books, may listen if their serviceman can be persuaded to talk about his battles, but they cannot feel the full force of the experience.

One young marine who saw the newsreel about the battle of Tarawa, in which he had taken part, wrote home to his parents, who had also seen it, that the picture was all right as far as it went. But, he wrote, "It didn't show the life blood of more than a thousand American boys draining away into the sea and the coral. You couldn't smell the cordite of the burning shells and the stink of death that hung heavily in the tropic air. Your ears didn't deafen for seventy-six hours because of the ceaseless cannonading, the screech of falling bombs, the staccato of machine gun and rifle fire. . . . The icy fingers of death didn't grip at your throat when the images flickered on the screen as they did at the throats of the marines who won the blood-drenched island. More than a thousand stout marine hearts beat their last. Boys went blind. Some lost arms, legs, feet, and hands. Some suffered disfiguring wounds that even the miracles of plastic surgery won't repair. Even those marines who spent seventy-six hours of hell on Tarawa without a single physical scratch have wounds seared deep in their souls . . ."

Such a battle is not the only wearing phase of combat. Someone has said, "War is long periods of boredom relieved by short periods of acute fear." War is mostly waiting — during the long weeks while the ship is enroute to its battle station, during the long hours it takes to fly to and from the "thirty seconds over Tokyo," during the long night before the attack at dawn.

Nor is this waiting a time of restful relaxation. It is waiting in tense dread of the ordeal ahead, waiting in the knowledge that tomorrow you may die, waiting in fear that you may fail in the awful test of action, waiting on the alert for the enemy fire that may come unexpectedly from ahead, above, or behind. It is upon the heels of such waiting that battle comes with its intolerable demands.

No wonder men crack under the strain of it. Men, big men with powerful bodies, burst into tears and cry for days. Men in the face of continuous bursts of flame are scared sightless, in the face of splintered shells are frightened speechless. Men jump out of foxholes, or go over the top to attack, raise their arms to throw a grenade and find them paralyzed—stiff, outstretched, frozen so with fear.

The sooner the better

These men, and the others whose symptoms are less spectacular—those who can't stop shaking, can't eat, can't sleep, can't get over their tortured dreams—are sometimes said to have war neurosis. Psychiatrists prefer to say the men have combat nerves, combat fatigue, war weariness, task-force fever, destroyer stomach, or any one of several other names, depending on the symptoms and the conditions under which the breakdown occurred. The soldiers themselves call it by more piquant names. If a man cracks in battle, he's "bomb happy." In Iceland or Greenland he's "glacier happy." If he's in an air crew in the South Pacific, he has an attack of Zero-itis.

Whether or not the symptoms constitute true psychoneurosis we may leave for the doctors to decide. The important point is that if these men can be given quick treatment, right at the front, the great majority of them recover and are able to return to duty.

The principle here is an old one. Everyone knows that if a rider falls from his horse, he should be made to mount again at once, so the fear caused by his accident does not become fixed into a fear of all horses and all riding. The first thing a pilot who cracks up but isn't hurt should do is go right back up as soon as possible. The longer he goes without flying again the harder it is for him to go back.

Similarly if the men who break down in battle are treated at once, within a few hours, they usually recover. If they are given rest, warm baths, sedatives if necessary, and above all a chance to talk over their difficulties with an understanding doctor, their emotion is lessened and the experience fades without leaving an aftermath of recurrent symptoms. The fear reaction does not become a fixed pattern.

Jack was one of the lucky ones in this respect. He was a tough army sergeant, an infantryman with the Purple Heart and a medal for valor, but he came in from the line one day crying like a baby, unable to stop it or to tell anyone why he was crying. The psychiatrist got hold of him, administered proper treatment, and the story came out.

During the battle Jack had to send someone to scout the position of the Jerries his men were supposed to clean out of their nest. He chose Nick. Halfway across the field a shell hit Nick and he fell. Jack rushed over "to save him," but Nick was dead. "He was my buddy," said Jack, "from my home town, and I sent him out to check those guns. I sent him to his death."

Quietly the doctor talked with Jack, got him to see that he had only been doing his job, as Nick had been doing his. It was bad luck but it was not Jack's fault that the shell hit Nick on that trip. The doctor's calm, his understanding and good sense, helped to allay Jack's feeling of guilt, and in a few days he returned to his post.

Ralph was not so lucky. He had been given a citation for gallantry in the North African campaign and another in the battle for the Anzio beachhead, so he was anything but a coward. Later in the Italian campaign he was making his way back to his own lines in the early dawn after a night at an observation post. A Nazi sniper began shooting at him and he took cover in a jeep that was stalled by the roadside. When he decided to leave a few minutes later, he found that both his arms were paralyzed. They were completely without feeling from the finger tips to the shoulders.

The doctor at the front, suspecting that Ralph was suffering from hysteria neurosis, sent him to a hospital behind the lines, and there the psychiatrist was able to achieve an apparent recovery. Enroute back to his outfit, though, Ralph was strafed by Nazi airplanes. Immediately his paralysis returned, and with it a complete inability to speak.

This time Ralph was evacuated to a hospital in the United States, and after two months of treatment was discharged considerably improved in the use of his arms and in his speech, though he still stuttered when he got excited.

He might have got over this in time, but fate seemed against him. Two months after his return home, his little girl was killed by a hit-and-run driver. Again Ralph's paralysis in arms and speech returned. The pattern of this response to strain was becoming fixed.

Who's to judge?

Most of us, if we make the effort to understand, can see how a man might break down in combat. We can see that battle conditions are so tough that the most normal individual might reach his breaking point. But most of the discharges for psychoneurosis occur during training, before the man has gone overseas or seen action at all. What about these men, whom the soldiers call "barrack wacky"? Are they weaklings?

Not necessarily so at all. Could you fairly call Tom the lawyer or Larry the accountant who is turning social worker a weakling? Of course not.

It is true that many of these men who break in camp reach their limit of endurance more quickly than others—just as some men come down with pneumonia or some other disease under training conditions, without having to wait for the fatigue and exposure of the foxhole and the beachhead. It is also true that more of the camp casualties than of the combat cases have a prewar history of neurotic behavior in some degree or form.

Each of us reacts to different pressures according to the responses he has learned, the habits he has formed. Some men with neurotic tendencies get through war without difficulty because its demands do not press on their particular sore spots. But put these men back under the strain of a nagging wife or of financial worries and they will go to pieces in their turn.

Every man has his own particular devil, or devils, and his own brand of hell. Put him in a situation — whether at home, in camp, or in combat — that arouses this devil and creates this hell, and he will develop a psychoneurosis. This being the case, who is to judge, saying that one who breaks down is a weakling while another is not?

Besides, combat conditions are not entirely remote from training. Thoughts about killing and being killed, with all the emotional conflicts they produce, can arise as well during target practice and the mock battles of training as in combat. The soldier who has an overly active imagination may have to endure in advance the torments of the front itself. Who of us has not found some dreaded ordeal less terrible in reality than it seemed in prospect?

In many cases it is the family and home that precipitate the man's breakdown. The wife perhaps finds that she can't make the furnace work, or balance the bank account, or take the mouse out of the trap. The fuse has blown out, the awful intricacies of the rationing system have increased, the roof leaks, and the baby is flushed and cross — measles probably. She pours out all these woes in her letters to her husband.

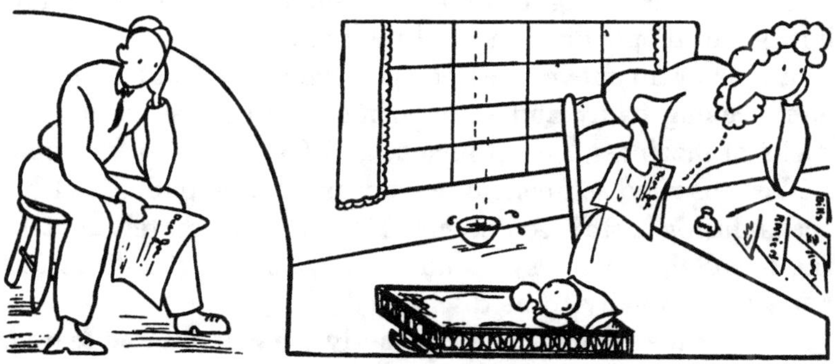

A double load

Stuck in an army camp, unable to go at once to her rescue as he always has in the past, the husband feels guilty and worried. In time, unless he rebels against such letters or unless his wife learns to stand on her own feet, the strain of a double responsibility — to his family at home and to his country at war — may prove more than he can carry successfully.

Sam's neurosis

Edith's husband Sam is one of those whose breakdown has occurred in anticipation of combat, though he was at the time overseas. Edith is mistaken in thinking that Sam's tendency to neurotic symptoms — anxiety, sweating, and vomiting — has not bothered him in the army. True, by virtue of his ability and hard work, he has risen from private to first lieutenant in a very short time. But he has done so, just as he got through his examinations at school, at the cost of considerable emotional strain.

When he was commissioned as an officer and sent overseas, he worried about how he would acquit himself in action. He was extremely conscious of his responsibility as an officer, felt that he must be a calm, aggressive leader, never showing fear or emotion of any kind before his men. But he was constantly afraid that something would happen beyond his control and he would be disgraced.

Outwardly, though, he got along all right. His superior officers liked him, thought him an able man. They did not know how his heart pounded most of the time.

As his outfit moved nearer and nearer the front, Sam began sleeping badly and suffered more and more often from spells of dizziness, sick stomach, and feelings of suffocation. At last his rigid self-control gave way, and he had one of his spells during a staff conference. He was immediately sent to the hospital, but his symptoms got worse instead of better, and he had finally to be discharged.

At no time could Sam say exactly what it was he feared. He was sure that he was no more afraid of dying than the next man, and no more likely to run away when confronted with the danger of death. Why, then, did he have this fear so intense that it incapacitated him for his job?

Sam was reacting to the coming test of battle just as he always had to examinations in school. Any impending situation that is a severe test of his abilities is to Sam what the bell was to Pavlov's dog or the gun to Tom the lawyer. Sam has acquired the habit of responding to such tests with sweating, vomiting, and a racing heart.

The early experiences that conditioned Sam in this way are lost to his conscious memory, but there are some suggestive facts in his personal history: as a child he was very fat; his parents are intelligent, proud, and ambitious; and his father at least is a nervous, irritable person. Perhaps during Sam's childhood these factors worked together in some such fashion as this.

Sam is teased and ridiculed as "fatties" usually are. When he wants to play baseball with the gang, he is pushed aside with the comment, "You couldn't run; you're too fat." But Sam wants very much to play, to be included in the gang. It occurs to him that if he had a catcher's mitt, which none of the others have, they would let him play. So he begs his parents to buy him one.

His father and mother see this as their chance. Being proud and ambitious and themselves given to intellectual pursuits, they are anxious that Sam should do exceptionally well in school. He's getting along well enough, but they're sure he could do much better if he tried harder. He has a final examination coming up, for which he has not been studying. So they tell him that if he gets the best grade in the class on this examination, they will buy him the catcher's mitt.

Sam, wanting that mitt more than he has ever wanted anything in his short life, gets down to work—his father all the while in his own tense, nervous way pointing out the major importance of this, that, and the other thing that Sam must learn.

As the day of the examination comes nearer, Sam feels desperate. He just *must* be able to answer every question so that nobody in the class can beat him, yet he can't possibly learn all the things his nervous, scolding father thinks he must know. He gets tense and tight with fear that he won't make the goal set for him; his head whirls, his heart pounds, he gets sick to his stomach and vomits.

But he answers every question on the examination. He leads the class, gets his mitt, is allowed to play with the gang. And he discovers that the boys who make fun of him on the baseball lot will admire him when he beats them in the classroom. At the same time his parents have found out how to make Sam measure up to their standards for him. So the whole process is repeated again and again—Sam's father urging him to more and more effort before each examination, Sam trying so hard he gets sick.

After a time he no longer needs the urging or the promise of some coveted reward. He has formed the habit of working to lead his class; everyone expects him to do so; and all the emotion originally attached to the catcher's mitt has been transferred to the examination itself. Sam no longer feels he must excel in order to get something he wants; he just feels he must excel. Even after experience has shown him that he can do things well, the behavior pattern of anxiety, dizziness, fast heart, and vomiting remains to plague him every time he faces a test of his ability to measure up to what is expected of him.

Naturally, Sam's symptoms did not improve when he was sent to the army hospital. What he has subconsciously feared since he was a child has come to pass. In his own eyes he has failed to measure up; he is being discharged as inadequate for this job. So he remains upset, his letters sound depressed and discouraged "and apologetic somehow, as though he had done something to be ashamed of."

If Sam wishes to get rid of these neurotic symptoms, he must come to understand what is causing them and then must apply himself to the task, not an easy one, of learning new responses to test situations. He must learn that failure comes to all men at some time in their lives, and that the failure to measure up is not itself so important as the way one stands up to it. He must learn not to care so much what others think of him, to relax a little the high standards to which he rigidly holds himself, to tolerate a reasonable degree of human frailty in himself.

No middle ground

In some cases the family's distress at the news of what has happened to their serviceman is intensified by the fact that he has been in the hospital. They naturally assume this means he is as sick as he would be if he went to the hospital at home. Relatively few psychoneurotic breakdowns are severe or complete enough to require hospitalization under ordinary circumstances, but circumstances are not ordinary in the military services.

If you or I get a spell of nervous jitters we can telephone the office or the factory, say we are not feeling well enough to work, and occupy ourselves at home until the spell has passed. We would not think of going to the hospital in such a case. But the military services have no homes for the men to rest in. A soldier or sailor or marine must be on active duty with all that this demands of him or he must be called sick and go to the hospital; there is no middle ground. So his being in the hospital does not mean that he is seriously or dangerously ill or that he will be an invalid when he comes home. He may be perfectly able to work most of the time.

But if he is able to work, you may ask, why is he not kept on duty in the army? Even though a man can work nineteen days out of twenty, the military authorities do not feel they dare take the chance of his being unable to do his job on the twentieth day. The risk to his own life and others' is too great if he is likely to be upset at a crucial moment. Besides, most such men will do better and be of greater service at home.

You need not be afraid, then, that your man will have to go to the hospital when he comes home. In the few cases where the men discharged for psychoneurosis are ill enough to need further hospital care, they will be transferred to a veterans' hospital or some similar institution. The others, the great majority, will be much better off out of the hospital.

Doctors have discovered that an active convalescence is much better than a passive one in almost every case. Even surgical patients or women after childbirth recover their strength much faster if they are not kept in bed too long. This is especially true of neurotics, who must not be allowed to brood over their memories and their failures. They should not be permitted to get the habit of being sick. There is something seductive about a bed; a person may learn to rely too much on its shelter and comfort, so that he does not want to leave it and face once more the problems and conflicts of the workaday world.

This is strikingly demonstrated by what happened to Homer. He had a bad time in the navy, though he went through seven big naval engagements without a scratch. Without a scratch on his body, that is, but he had wounds just the same, wounds to his nerves, and these did not heal very well. He was in the naval hospital for some time, sullen, so depressed he would not talk, unable to keep any food on his stomach, tortured with nightmares about bombs falling on his ship.

Then the doctors tried a daring experiment. They asked Homer to go with some other men on a tour of armament factories, talking to the workers about the war and the great need for more ammunition. Homer didn't like the idea much but he really didn't care enough one way or the other to say no. If they thought he was in shape to make such a trip, he'd try it.

The first few days he was as sullen and closemouthed as ever. He would give his little talk when it was time, but when it was over he was glad to be quiet and alone again.

Then he began to change. "I began to warm up," he said. "I began to feel better when people came up after my talk, shook my hand, and told me they were grateful for what I'd done for them. That was a new line. They talked as though they thought I'd been a hero. And I'd been thinking I was a washout.

"Meeting those people that way, finding they didn't think I was nuts, began to get me. The longer the trip lasted, the more people I met, and the more of those fine dinners they gave us, the better I felt. Now all that's the matter with me is that I run out of push, get tired too easily. But I guess I'll get over that too before long."

What help there is

Because most of these men are able to be up and at work doesn't mean they would not benefit by good psychiatric care. If their disability is service-connected, they are entitled to receive such care at the outpatient clinics of the veterans' hospitals. But the number of such mental hospitals is limited, so that many discharged veterans will not live near enough to one to take advantage of its services. Besides, these hospitals are already overcrowded and their staffs are greatly overworked.

It is certainly to be hoped that either the federal government or the various local communities will provide, as a few have done, good psychiatric or mental hygiene clinics to which these men can go for the advice and treatment they need. Until such clinics are established, however, it will be up to the men themselves and their families to secure what help is necessary.

They can engage the services of a good psychiatrist in private practice, if one is available and they can afford to pay his fees. Unfortunately, however, there are only some three thousand trained psychiatrists in the whole United States and their fees are the high ones of most medical specialists.

Your family doctor, though he has not had special training in nervous and mental disorders, can be of great help nonetheless. His difficulty will be in sparing enough time and in overcoming his habit of making little explanation. The nervous patient needs a good deal of time, so that he can talk easily and freely about his difficulties, and he needs a lot of explanation about what is causing those difficulties and what he can do about them. He must be made to understand his fears and be given the heart to fight against them, and this takes a good deal more than a few lines of writing on a prescription pad. If the doctor's purpose is to get the patient well, he will only defeat that purpose by acting on his usual assumption that he is the only one who needs to know what is wrong with the patient.

Good advice is to be had too from the psychiatric social workers employed by the Red Cross and other social agencies in your community. You need have no hesitation about seeking their help; they are glad to give it and are in their offices for this very purpose. And they are much better qualified by training and experience to advise you wisely than is your aunt, your next-door neighbor, or your bridge-club friend.

What he needs

With the best of advice from a psychiatrist, the family doctor, or a psychiatric social worker, the psychoneurotic may still fall short in his recovery unless his folks at home, his friends, and his social and business associates play their part wisely and well. In the end the sick man must fight his own way back to health, but he cannot do it in the face of indifference, impatience, or active antagonism on the part of those closest to him. Genuine kindness from his family and the community will be his best psychologic medicine. He does not want and will not benefit from sentimental sympathy, but wise and kindly understanding will greatly ease his road back to health.

What he needs most is to get back his faith in life and in himself, in his own ability to work and play and live like other people. To help him most, then, is to give him a chance for satisfying work, pleasure, and love, to help him find a job, make friends, and have fun.

Under such a regime the symptoms that trouble him will lessen and disappear with time—the length of time depending upon their severity and on how long he has had them. If their onset was sudden and recent, they will probably disappear sooner than if they developed gradually long before he went into military service. But whatever their duration, while he has them he, and you with him, must learn to live with them—just as Betty and Dick must learn to live with the fact of Dick's missing arm.

Perhaps, as we have said, his trouble is so slight that it will interfere with his life no more than a missing finger would. But if the handicap is more severe than that, face it; don't ignore it, pretending it doesn't exist. Just such pretense is often part of the psychoneurotic's trouble. He refuses to admit even to himself that he has any handicap whatever, drives himself harder and harder, gets tenser and tenser, until he crosses the threshold of his endurance and breaks down.

Your serviceman has discovered, if he did not know it before, that certain symptoms will appear when he meets a certain problem or kind of strain. You expect this to be less true as time goes on, but in the meantime recognize its presence, decide what difference it should make in your lives, and plan accordingly. Then forget it as much and as often as you can.

At times it can't be forgotten of course; cold sweat, dizziness, diarrhea, and vomiting, for instance, are obvious symptoms that cannot be entirely ignored. But they can be accepted as symptoms, just as headache from eyestrain or pain from a sprained ankle can be accepted as symptoms, and dealt with when they occur. If the symptoms are not fussed over, magnified into a major disaster, or cultivated as alibis, they will return less often and less severely.

Remember that these symptoms, whether mental or physical, are not the neurosis but its manifestations. They will come and go until the underlying personality disorder that produces them has been corrected. Psychoneurosis is more like malaria than, say, pneumonia. One does not have it once and then is done with it. Its acute attacks recur until the patient is rid of the underlying cause. The spells of nervousness and anxiety will appear from time to time, lasting for an hour, a day, or a week, but they will pass. They will be less unpleasant and will pass more quickly if they are taken as easily as possible.

Take it easy

Sleeplessness is a good example. It is unpleasant not to be able to drop off to sleep when one goes to bed. But to get upset about it, turn and toss, punch the pillow this way and that, and work up a good fit of temper about it, only aggravates the situation, pushing sleep farther and farther away.

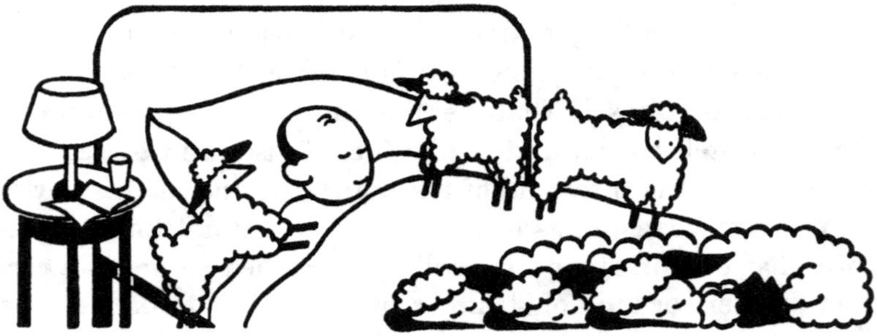

The slowdown for sleep

Sleep won't come because the mind is too keyed up to quit working. So the helpful measures are those that slow down the mental processes, not those that stir them up.

Let the man who worries about sleeping try starting the slowdown about two hours before he plans to go to bed—with quiet music, an hour of quiet reading on some pleasant subject, some lazy talk about unexciting things. Then a warm bath perhaps, a glass of hot milk, and to bed. Not to *try* to go to sleep; trying hard will only wake him up. Let him lie comfortably relaxed, all his muscles, even those of the eyes and jaws, gone slack and loose, his mind at rest in the sure knowledge—for this is the truth—that it doesn't really matter whether he sleeps or not as long as he rests.

The tiring effects of sleeplessness come not half so much from the lack of sleep itself as from the restless twisting and turning, fussing and stewing with which people fight it. The value of devices such as counting sheep lies in their calming monotony. Repeating a few lines of poetry or a Bible verse over and over, thinking each word slowly and gently, has the same effect, so long as the mind does not dart off to the worries and anxieties of the day before or the day approaching. Sleep comes to a slow, relaxed mind, not to an active, angry, worried one.

This same quiet refusal to be disturbed is the best way to deal with any neurotic symptom; it will not long withstand it. Whereas fighting it angrily and rebelliously only makes it stronger.

One of the symptoms most difficult to endure calmly is the particular kind of fear to which the neurotic may be subject. It is a kind of terror that may come over him when he least expects it; it may wake him from a sound sleep. Unless this is checked quickly it will spread in his mind to a feeling of panic so overwhelming that he is paralyzed into inaction. He is literally too afraid to move.

To head off the panic and keep the fear within reasonable bounds he should immediately try to focus it upon its cause. He may say to himself, "Last night I was not afraid. What has happened since then to make me feel this fear?"

The answer will probably be that nothing has happened, that there is no more cause for fear now than there was yesterday. But yesterday he was busy at work with his mind full of other things. Then the thing to do now is to occupy himself with something else. The best thing is for him to try to analyze the fear itself, forcing himself to put it into actual words, writing it out on paper if necessary.

Exactly what is it that he fears? He must not let himself be satisfied with a vague and formless answer, such as "I'm afraid of the future." Precisely what in the future? That his mother will die, that the house will burn down, that he will lose his job?

In most cases he will find that he cannot name any specific thing he is afraid of, and this discovery, plus the exercise itself, will go far toward dispelling the emotion that has got hold of him.

If he can pin his fear to one namable cause, he has something to work on. Suppose he is afraid that he will lose his job. Why does he think so? Are his facts sufficient grounds for the fear? What can he do about them? If he does lose his job, what exactly will be the effects? What steps can he take toward finding another job? And so on. By the time he has worked out a possible course of action, most of his fear will be gone.

One specter that haunts many neurotics is the fear that they are losing or will lose their minds. Since something is out of order in their mental processes, they jump to the conclusion that they're going insane. This fear is unfounded. Psychoneurosis is not likely to develop into psychosis, any more than chicken pox becomes smallpox. Sometimes, it is true, a person who has had chicken pox will contract smallpox, but many psychiatrists think this is unlikely in mental illness. They believe that a person who breaks down neurotically will always react to strain in that way, never with a psychosis.

New habits for old

The mental conflict or personality disorder that lies at the root of a neurotic's difficulty is such an individual matter that it must be left to the psychiatrist working with his patient. If the cause is a faulty habit pattern, the treatment can only be a form of re-education. The patient has learned his habitual responses by practicing them over a long period of years. If he wishes to replace them with less disturbing responses, he must learn these new habits in the same way: by regular, consistent practice.

This learning process is neither easy nor speedy. The man cannot simply say "I will be different" and presto! wake up the next morning a new person. His learned response has become automatic with constant practice, just as shifting gears at the proper time has become automatic for an experienced driver, and the automatic emotional response will be the line of least resistance, much easier than taking conscious thought to apply the desired new approach.

The patient attempting to change his personality habit patterns will often get discouraged and think it can't be done. He must remember that the old way of reacting has been in the saddle for twenty or thirty years; it cannot be unseated without some effort. The patient and his neurosis are friendly enemies. Each time he reacts to a situation with a spell of nerves, the point is one for the neurosis; each time he meets a crisis calmly, however minor a one, the score goes to the person he wants to become: a healthier, happier, more relaxed person.

Perhaps we can make this process clearer by applying it to the habit of worrying that is so common among neurotics. Worry is pointless thinking; it moves in circles, never in a straight line toward any real solution. Often the psychoneurotic has learned to use this fruitless method of approach to every event or problem he meets. If he wishes to substitute a better method, he must first check up on the importance of the things he worries about. Doing this honestly will force him to admit that most of them are not worth a minute's thought, let alone the hours' reviewing he gives them. What does it matter if the bus driver was discourteous yesterday? Or if the boss did bawl him out for being late this morning? Or if his wife's accounts are a dollar or so out of balance?

If the problem is a real one involving a major decision, let him pick a time when he is relatively calm and free from other concerns, sit down with pencil and paper, and write out all the possible courses of action he has to choose among. Then list the advantages and disadvantages of each. In full recognition of the fact that no one of them will suit him perfectly, he should make the best decision he can on the basis of whatever evidence he has. Then he must try to forget the whole matter until it is time to act on his decision.

At first his mind will go back to the problem again and again. That is his old way. Each time this happens he asks himself, Have I any new evidence to be considered? No. Then the decision still stands; I will not think about it. Each time he succeeds in putting it out of his mind, the old habit is loosened and the new one strengthened. And once his decision has been put into effect, he must recognize that time and energy spent in futile regrets for the courses of action he turned down is simply crying over spilled milk, which is only another form of worrying.

Whenever a man who is trying to rid himself of the worry habit finds himself caught in its circle, he must immediately break out of it somehow, anyhow. He can turn on the radio, pick up an interesting book, go to a movie. His goal is eventually to achieve the orderly thinking described by Bertrand Russell in *The Conquest of Happiness*: "The wise man thinks about his troubles only when there is some purpose in doing so; at other times he thinks of other things. . . . It is amazing how much both happiness and efficiency can be increased by the cultivation of an orderly mind, which thinks about a matter adequately at the right time rather than inadequately at all times."

Perhaps the first thing most victims of psychoneurosis need to learn is to accept their limitations—to keep their eye upon what they *have* rather than upon what they *haven't.* So very often their basic conflict is between their desires and their attainments, between what they are and what they would like to be.

Imagine a middle-aged ditch digger of great brawn but limited education being discontented because he isn't a college professor; or a girl who isn't beautiful, who can't act,

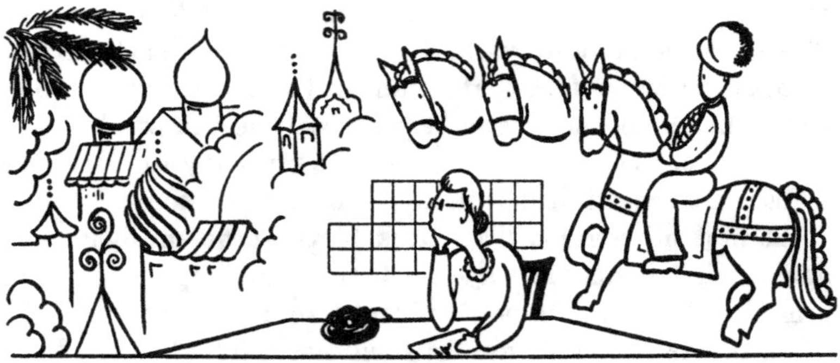

Keep your dreams within reason

can't dance, can't sing, making herself unhappy with longings for the fame and fortune of a movie star. The futility of their desires is obvious, because the gap is so wide between what they want and what they can possibly have. Yet many, many people spoil their lives with longings just as futile but not so obviously so.

Ambition is a useful character trait, but it becomes a threat to mental health when it drives a person toward a goal that is too far beyond his reach.

Again the job's the thing

"To be useful is the most constructive aid to being self-respecting, and a completely self-respecting person is usually in good mental health." If the psychoneurotic serviceman has suffered a blow to his self-respect because of his breakdown, he needs above everything else to feel useful and productive again. That is, he needs a job.

In some cases he may have to take it easy for a while and begin his return to work with a job less demanding than he formerly had or than he expects eventually to have again. This was the case with Bob. Before the war he worked for a publishing company selling magazines and made a good living at it. And, as he said, "If you can make a living in that line, you're a *salesman,* brother."

In the army he was assigned to an armored division and was among the first troops landed in Africa. Things were tough. Three times Bob was the sole survivor in a tank accident, all his crewmates being burned to death or blown to pieces each time. After his third experience of this kind, Bob went to pieces and was discharged for anxiety neurosis.

His condition improved gradually and he wanted to get back to work, but he knew he had not recovered enough of his old punch and self-confidence to make a go of his magazine selling. On that job he sometimes had to work ten and twelve hours a day; now he is tired out at the end of eight. So under the guidance of employment counselors, he decided to take a course in bookkeeping and get a job in that line until he is stronger. It will be quiet and will require less emotional strain and physical energy.

Bob knows he is a better salesman than clerical worker, and he fully expects to go back to selling again someday. In the meantime he will be busy, earning his own way, and much happier than just sitting around at home.

The question that bothers many of these men, of course, is whether they can find a job. Will employers hire them when they have an N-P discharge? With relatively few exceptions, the answer is definitely yes.

It is true that some employers, uninformed along with the rest of the public, have been afraid to hire men with any record of mental illness. But they are getting over this rapidly, because of experiences like that of the man who was persuaded by an employment service to hire an N-P for a job he badly needed done. He hired the man, he said, against his better judgment. Three weeks later he called the employment service. "Hey, have you got any more men like that. N-P or not, he's the best worker I've got in the whole place."

Employers who have made it a policy not to hire any N-P are not only being very unfair to the individual, but they are depriving themselves of good employees. They will do well to remember that the neurotic is usually the overconscientious kind of person who drives himself hard. The difficulty, if there is any, will be to keep him from working too hard. As someone has said, "The world's best work is done by nervous people." It is only ignorance not to understand that a man may be unfit for military service and yet perfectly able to fill any number of civilian jobs very well.

What makes the attitude of these few employers foolish is that they already have a goodly number of psychoneurotics on their payrolls, and among them very likely are some of their ablest executives. It is estimated that at least twenty-five per cent of any large working organization is made up of neurotic, maladjusted individuals. The only difference is that the veteran comes home with a name for his maladjustment; the civilian neurotic just hasn't been diagnosed and labeled.

Making the most of the veteran's abilities requires proper placement, of course, just as it does in the case of the physically handicapped and, for the best results, with the normal worker. (See pages 93 to 94.) The proper kind of job is essential for anyone's mental health. The reports of psychiatric studies in industry tell many stories of employees who were doing bad work and suffering emotional upsets because they were placed in the wrong kind of job.

Progressive employers are seeing to it that their personnel officers are trained in mental hygiene, that they know enough about psychology and mental illness to recognize and deal with symptoms of emotional disturbance before it reaches the breakdown stage. When an employee comes to such a trained officer and says "I just can't stand the noise in there," the officer will know better than to dismiss him with a casual "Oh, you're all right, John. That noise isn't so bad." He will know that though the noise doesn't seem so bad to *him,* it may be hell for the man whose nerves have been left edgy by the din of the battlefield. A veteran who still is oversensitive to noise may be able to stand the hum of motors all right, but he ought not to be placed in a job where he will be subject to sudden, sharp noises such as the clanging of steel or loud bells or whistles.

Nor should a nervous man be loaded with responsibilities. Start him out with a job that isn't too demanding and ease him gradually into the more exacting positions. But don't give him a night watchman's job in the mistaken idea that it is just right because it's light work. Its loneliness and time for thought are the very things he should not have. He needs pleasant and continuous occupation for his mind as well as his hands.

Above all, don't expect a veteran to do well in a job that is marked by long periods of slack work punctuated with peaks of rush and bustle. This is precisely the kind of thing that got him down in the armed forces.

The wise employer will pay more attention to an applicant's prewar record than to his illness in the army. If he was steady and reliable in the jobs he held before the war, then with proper placement and a little time for adjustment he will be a valuable employee again.

The man with seizures

There is a special problem involved in the employment of men who are subject to epileptic seizures. Epilepsy is not a psychoneurosis, but it is a nervous affliction from which many veterans may suffer, so a few words about it are in order.

Epilepsy is very common among us; some half a million persons in the United States alone are subject to seizures. And the number will be greater after the war because injuries to the brain may produce the attacks and the strain of military life may lower the threshold of endurance in those who have any predisposition to the disease.

Many persons have epileptic seizures so slight and short that no one is aware of them, not even the person himself sometimes. He may just stop short in the middle of the sentence, blink his eyes a few times, and go on with what he was saying. Those who suffer from more severe attacks may lose consciousness, fall, and twitch or shake violently. They may be unusually flushed or abnormally pale, and saliva may collect on their lips.

A severe convulsion of this kind is not pleasant to see, and from this fact in part has come the mistaken and very unfair idea that epilepsy is a horrible and shameful disease—an attitude that adds so much heartbreak to the epileptic's handicap.

Epileptics usually have perfectly normal minds; indeed many of them are above average in intelligence and accomplishment. Many of the world's great men have been epileptics: Julius Caesar for one, and also Swinburne the poet, Paganini the violinist, Maupassant the writer, and Van Gogh the painter.

The epileptic patient must have competent and experienced medical care, but with this in the vast majority of cases the attacks can be greatly reduced in number and severity. The patient himself, of course, must take reasonable precautions. He ought not, for instance, to drive a car, run an elevator, or work with moving machinery. Beyond such necessary allowances for his handicap, he should live a full and rounded life. He needs to keep busy, to enjoy stimulating companionship and recreation, and to cultivate a variety of interesting hobbies.

In this all-important matter of keeping his morale high, the cooperation of his family and friends is vital. Shame and anxiety are contagious. Horror and fear in those around him will only add to his distress and his inclination to withdraw from people, which is one of the worst things he can do. His family must encourage him and foster his self-confidence, but they should not be too solicitous or protective. He should be given every possible freedom of decision and action compatible with reasonable precautions for his safety.

There is no reason, except uninformed public opinion and practice, to prevent the epileptic from living a happy and useful life or from holding a useful and satisfying job.

This makes it all the more unfortunate that in America most employers will not hire a confessed epileptic and a seizure occurring on the job is considered a cause for discharge. In this we are inexcusably backward. After all, is it not stupid, as well as unjust, to deny employment to a qualified worker just because for a few minutes each week or month or year he may present a distressing appearance?

Public education on this whole matter is badly needed. And it would help to solve the employment problem if the existing workmen's compensation laws were changed to permit an epileptic to work at his own risk. At present the employer is liable for any injury that occurs to him while he is at work. However, much of the danger of injury could be removed by proper job placement. The epileptic ought not to be placed in a job where his occasional and temporary loss of consciousness could endanger his life or another's.

There is more information on this important subject and

more helpful advice for the epileptic's family and friends in the books on the reading list that follows this chapter. Or you may write for information to either of these national organizations: the American Epilepsy League, 50 State Street, Boston, Massachusetts; the Association to Control Epilepsy, 22 East Sixty-seventh Street, New York City.

Beware of a cushion

Perhaps the problem of jobs for psychoneurotic veterans does not seem important to you. Are they not entitled to pensions? you ask. Well, are they?

The question is easy to answer in the case of a man with no prewar history of neurotic tendencies who cracks in combat. But what about the man who has a long history of such difficulties and who breaks down in training? His breakdown is just as real, but is it service-connected?

An army doctor who has had a good deal to do with the treatment of men who break under the strain of training as plane pilots has told something of his heartbreaking experience when he accompanies some of these men to their homes. It is his job to explain to the parents what kind of care they must give the man to restore him to normal usefulness. And the parents are always resentful. "He was perfectly healthy when you began on him," they say. "But now look what you've done to him."

Sam's parents might say this too, or his wife Edith. But would it be the truth? Did the army or the war produce Sam's breakdown? When he has been suffering from exactly the same trouble ever since he was a child?

Or what about a case like Rodney's? Rodney came to the army doctors complaining of severe pains in his back and legs. They could find nothing physically wrong with him, so they investigated his prewar history. They learned that he had never got on well at school, that each time he got into a scrape his parents took him out of that school and put him in another. Finally they allowed him to quit school and go to work.

He didn't get on in jobs either. But his father was an influential man and always came to his rescue when he got into trouble. If he got arrested for careless driving, his father paid his fines. If he was broke, his father gave him money to tide him over until the next payday. Actually it didn't much matter whether he worked or not.

With a history like this before them, the army doctors did not have much trouble understanding what was wrong with Rodney. In the army he was on his own. He no longer had his father's protection when things went wrong. He had always been able to get his own way by becoming depressed or angry. Here no one paid any attention to him when he sulked. The experience was so new to him that he had no way to meet it. He got upset, and his emotion was expressing itself in the pains that had sent him to the doctors.

Obviously Rodney was not suited to military service and had to be discharged. But was his disability service-connected? The majority opinion is no. Only about twenty per cent of all psychoneurotic disabilities have been rated as incurred in the line of military duty.

Whatever the rating given your serviceman, do not let him worry about the size of his pension or the absence of any at all. It could be his greatest obstacle to recovery. Because of the nature of his illness, such a cushion is more dangerous even for him than for one physically handicapped like Dick. It would be difficult for even the most normal person to get well if he were being paid to remain sick.

Don is a veteran of World War I whose trouble has been a neurotic fear of people. To leave his home, get on and off the streetcar, and work with people in any number was more than he could manage. So he was given a pension of one hundred dollars a month. He took a room with a kindly woman who looked after him as one might a child.

Then a neighbor of hers decided this was just making an old man of Don. If his fear wasn't catered to so much, he would be a lot better off. She told him so, and under her influence he overcame his fear enough to go to and from his brother's cigar store every afternoon, to help out because his brother was short of help.

Don was feeling very good about this until someone warned him that if he kept on this way, the Veterans Administration would decide he was able to work, and then he would lose his pension. This threat was enough to undo all the friendly neighbor had accomplished. Don enjoyed his greater freedom and the daily trips away from his lonely room, but he had come to depend on his pension and he was afraid to try to get along without it.

Until we find some way to provide a disabled veteran with the support he needs without compensating him for holding fast to his illness, don't be too upset if your man is not rated pensionable. It may well be the best thing that could happen to him.

Some do's and don'ts

Look to your own behavior. If you want to help your psychoneurotic serviceman, you will need to keep a careful watch on your own behavior and call often on your self-control. He may not be easy to live with. It is difficult for a healthy person to be patient with one whose nerves are sick. Why can't he sit still for a single minute? Why must he fuss so over such trifles? Why on earth doesn't he make up his mind and be done with it?

The answer is, he can't help it. He must and will learn to do so, but in the meantime, you, being the healthy one, must curb your own temper, your own nerves, your own irritability.

A man's family can get on his nerves perhaps quicker than anyone else, if they sigh and coax, or make themselves too busy in his behalf, or show their anxiety about his future. And few men, let alone neurotics, can long endure a nagging, scolding woman, or one whose tongue is never still. Let him enjoy some peace, some moments of silence, free from chatter, or you will force him to feel like the Irishman who wrote for his wife's tombstone:

Here lies a woman, no man can deny it;
She dies in peace, although she lived unquiet.
Her husband prays, if you this way should walk,
You will tread softly, for if she wakes she'll talk.

The most helpful wife or mother is calm, patient, and jolly. She makes home a cheerful place, easy to be comfortable in. This is much more important than perfect order or shining dustlessness. She sees to it, too, that mealtime is the occasion for shared jokes, good times, and hearty laughter, not for bickering, recriminations, and disciplining the children. "Whistle while you eat" is a good health rule for anyone and especially for the neurotic.

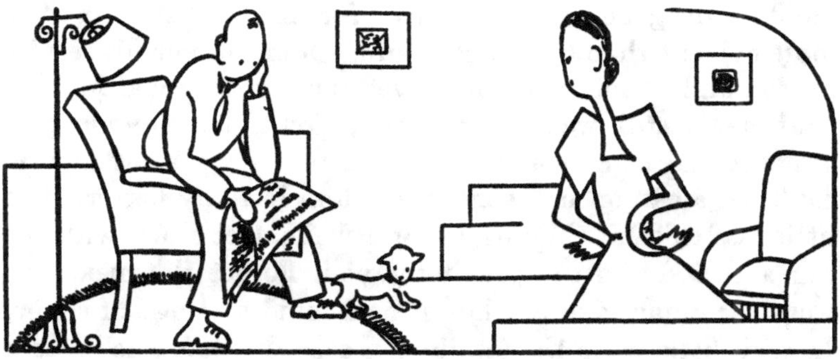

She lived unquiet!

All this is not only for the good of the nervous head of the house. It is a wise precaution against the children's learning unhealthy behavior patterns by imitation.

Don't lecture him; show him. If you try to carry out any of the suggestions that follow by means of little sermons or wordy advice, you will fail to achieve their purpose and yours. Your help must be indirect, for though he needs it, he is likely to resent it if he recognizes it as such.

Above all do not be constantly seeking credit for your help by pointing it out. If he is sure he can't eat dinner and then is lured into doing so by the tasty dishes you've concocted, don't say, "See, you ate that." Just cook some more good food tomorrow night. If he says he doesn't want to see people, yet enjoys himself when the friends you've invited come to play cards, don't ask, "Now that wasn't so bad, was it?" Just invite them in again sometime. Actions still speak louder than words, and they do more good.

Help him regain his self-respect. Many a man returning home with a discharge for psychoneurosis will suffer severely from feelings of shame, guilt, and failure. If your husband or son or brother is one of these, the first and major step in his recovery will be to regain his self-respect, and this will not be easy for him in the face of uninformed public opinion. You can help by making him feel that you have not lost your respect for him or your confidence in him. Let your pride in his abilities, his good looks, his knack for this or that, be a little more evident than before. Encourage him to wear his service button and to mix with other veterans on an equal footing.

If he is still weak and shaky, don't flaunt your own strength. Hearing you boast, "I'm not a weak sister who can't get a can open," won't make him feel any better. Be a little less efficient than usual for a while. Get stuck with the can and ask him to open it for you. Forget the meat you want for dinner and ask him if he'd mind getting it for you. In such little ways the family can ease the man back into a feeling of being useful.

Don't laugh; it isn't funny. The nervous veteran who dives under the restaurant table when a waiter drops a tray, whose hand shakes, or who can't keep the tears back when he's tired is very embarrassed by his actions. Don't laugh at him, and don't feel you have to make any comment unless he does. Pass over the incident with a quiet, reassuring nod. If he chooses to speak of it, let him know you take it as a matter of course and think nothing of it.

If you find it hard to understand, think a minute of what it means. He has learned to duck automatically for cover at every sharp noise, because where he's come from such noise means a bomb or a shell or the near presence of an enemy bent on killing. With the ducking goes a tightening of every nerve in fear of deadly danger. When he has had a sufficient spell of the safety you have enjoyed all along, his nerves and muscles will forget their pattern of response to danger and he won't have to duck any more.

Curb your curiosity. Don't ask a man why he isn't in uniform or where and how long he was in service. It really is none of your business, and you may be stirring up a feeling of inferiority that he is trying hard to overcome.

Don't ask him either how many Germans or Japs he killed. He may have killed as a matter of duty but he probably isn't proud of the fact. A feeling of guilt on this score may be partly to blame for his illness. In any case he is not likely to feel like boasting of his score as if the men he shot were clay pigeons in a skeet-shooting match. And in this he is to be congratulated over the person who asks the question.

Be a good listener. Do not nag, coax, and prod him into telling you about his experiences. Instead give him a chance to talk, and by your comfortable, casual manner try to make him feel like it. Perhaps after days of silence the urge to pour out his story will come upon him in the middle of the night. Listen quietly then, without comments or questions.

Talking it all out should give him some relief. Inability to share their troubles and fears is often a factor in the neurotics' illness; they bottle everything up to boil inside them. Talking it out to someone else releases the pent-up excitement and dissipates the tension. As we have seen, painful memories that are pushed into the subconscious mind may become serious troublemakers later. So let him talk if and when he can.

However, once he has talked it out, he should try to forget it. Do not encourage him to go on reliving again and again the horrors of it all. He may be too much inclined, as many neurotics are, to linger in the past, to mull over failures and dwell on might-have-beens. He must try to learn that these things that trouble him are past and gone. He cannot undo them, but he can make the present and the future what he will. He must not let what has happened become a stumbling block for him, as it has for the civilian neurotic who turns down a good job because he can't forget how he failed in the last one, who won't go to a dance because he made a social blunder the last time.

Avoid the sore spots. Try to discover what particular strains and stresses bring on his symptoms. Then as far as is practicable arrange your lives to be free of them. If climbing makes him jittery, hire someone else to put on the window screens and shingle the roof. If the responsibilities of a host excite him so that he can't sleep, don't fill your home with dinner guests five nights a week. If he's no good at figures, so that balancing the budget upsets his digestion for a week, quietly take over that task yourself. Work toward eliminating his nervous tensions, but in the meantime don't rub him where it hurts.

Don't argue over minor issues. He is quite likely to be unreasonably irritable. A perfectly harmless remark or ordinary incident may provoke him to an outburst of anger so uncalled-for that it will astonish everyone, including him. Don't argue about whatever caused the outburst; you will only pour oil on the fire. You can't reason about something that isn't reasonable. Just listen, letting the angry words go in one ear and out the other. Tell yourself what is perfectly true: This isn't the man I know talking; this is his sick nerves at work.

Let him alone when he's in a black mood. His moods are not just the ordinary spells of blues that all of us have from time to time. They are deeper and more brooding. They hang over him like a heavy cloud, robbing him for the moment of all life's satisfactions and hope. He wants to crawl away like a wounded animal, away even from those he loves.

Don't be alarmed if your man suffers from such moods; they will pass and in time he will feel better. Above all, don't take his moods personally, thinking that something you have said or done has offended him and brought them on. They come without any apparent reason and are a phase of his illness. After a while they will be less frequent and severe.

Don't magnify the importance of his symptoms. He may tend to do so. Especially if they take the form of physical pain, they provide an evident and acceptable cause for what ails him. But if he has been thoroughly examined by a competent doctor and pronounced physically sound, then accept the doctor's verdict. Don't think his fast and irregular heart means he is in danger of sudden death or that his stomach distress requires a special diet. Concentrate on getting his emotions under control and his way of living more normal and the symptoms will in time take care of themselves.

Don't, though, fall into the opposite error of dismissing his complaints as imaginary. You have no trouble seeing that he is not imagining the vomiting, the diarrhea, or the palpitating heart. Neither is he imagining the pain, the dizziness, the fear, or the depression that you can't see.

Don't talk about him when he is present. Don't say to a visitor in his hearing, "Johnny isn't feeling at all well this morning," or "Tim slept very badly last night," or "Al is having *such* a time with his nerves." This sort of thing is as bad for him as it is for children. It increases his self-consciousness, makes his illness a source of pleasure (we all like to be the subject of the conversation, whatever the pretext), and fixes his mind on his trouble instead of diverting it. If you must talk about him to others, do it when he isn't around.

Don't coddle him. As far as possible treat him like a well person. There is no more disgrace in having psychoneurosis than in having pneumonia, but there is no more virtue either. The aim in pneumonia is to get well as fast as possible; the aim in psychoneurosis is to get back to more healthy living as fast as possible. The fact that the neurotic's restlessness, irritability, moodiness, and the like constitute a real illness does not mean that he is to be excused from all effort to control them. He must try to get well again. So with your patient, understanding acceptance of his illness you must mix a gentle insistence on his gradual return to reasonableness, stability, and healthy activity. At the same time—

Do not expect too much of him too soon. He may be suffering from the kind of neurosis that makes the decision as to whether he will wash the car or mow the lawn as exhausting for him as a day's shopping or entertaining is for you. Perhaps visiting with his old friends steps up the machinery in his mind to such a point that he will be worn out at the end of half an hour. It may tax his emotional strength to read the newspaper, listen to a play on the radio, hear someone practicing on the piano.

He will learn in time to tolerate these things again, but he will have to do it gradually, in small doses at first. If the ticking of the clock bothers him at night, let him try patiently to hear it for just ten minutes, concentrating on the sound it makes and telling himself all the while that it is just the clock ticking. Then put it away until the following night, when he can try listening to it for a little longer period. After a week or two of such effort, the ticking will no longer bother him.

Don't push him when he's tired and upset. This is not the time for reaching decisions or making plans. Wait until he is feeling calm and rested. He will do the job better and more easily. General Montgomery once said, "I am never anxious when I fight my battles. If I am anxious, I don't fight them. I wait till I am ready." If he could afford to wait till the right time for action, so can most of us.

Strive to better his sense of proportion — and your own. The neurotic is oppressed by "the terrible importance of unimportant things." He wastes mental energy on trifles, fussing about things that do not matter. They are not trifles to him of course. He cannot accept the fact that most of his mountains are molehills, that most of the bridges he so dreads he will never have to cross. He takes everything, including himself, much too seriously. He can't laugh at himself with the author of this little verse:

> My work just worried me today
> So that I could not do my best,
> Until I had this lovely thought:
> The world can stand it if I rest.

This is a personality pattern, and it is not easy to change it. He must try to stand off and look at himself and his affairs as he might those of another. Are these things he frets about really important? Must those papers be on the boss's desk tomorrow morning however late he has to work tonight? Will he really be disgraced if he can't afford to paint the house till next year? Does it really make him any less a man that he can't tinker with his own car or make a garden grow like John Jones across the street?

He will never, of course, be able to *act* on the honest answers to such questions as long as his family prods his discontent. Why can't we have a garden like the Jones's? Just look how much money the Joneses save by John's fixing his own car. Of course if you earned as much as John Jones, we could have our house painted too. His wife's ambition to keep up with the Joneses has driven many a man into a neurosis.

Encourage him to face his problems. He is likely to want to run away from them. If the bank is threatening to foreclose the mortgage on the house, it is unpleasant to have to sit down and figure out exactly what to do about it. Ill-equipped as he is at the moment to deal with such a problem, he may want to let things drift, vaguely hoping they will work themselves out somehow. In the meantime he may try to escape the shadow that's hanging over him by resort to too much alcohol, the use of drugs, too much idle daydreaming, or angry tirades against the bank.

This too is a personality pattern, and not a healthy one. If he is to replace it with a sounder one, he must learn to face each unpleasantness, however small, and deal with it immediately and decisively. He may not like the action he must take—telling the grocer he can't pay the bill this month, firing an inefficient employee, asking the tenant to pay his overdue rent—but he will find himself greatly relieved to have acted, and he will not need such psychological crutches as alcohol and fantasy.

Guard him against gloomy self-pity. The psychoneurotic

habitually wears blue glasses. He sees nothing in his life to be gay about, is sure he is worse off than anyone else, and forever bewails the hand that fate has dealt him. He hears other people laugh occasionally and wonders how they do it; he envies them the happiness that he feels has been denied him.

In part at least this is the result of a romantic notion that happiness is some continuous state of untroubled bliss that comes to one as a gift from the gods. It isn't. The happiest people among us are often so in spite of the bad hand life has dealt them. All of us have troubles; all of us have spells of the blues when we wonder whether life is worth the effort. We have limitations we resent, dreams we can't make come true. But most of us have a capacity for taking pleasure in little satisfactions that the neurotic seems to lack. He walks alone, feeling misunderstood, without friends, having no one to sympathize with him, no one to love him. Or that's how it seems to him.

If he is to break this pattern he must work at being happy. He must learn that when a situation can't be changed, he has the choice of bemoaning it or of finding something in it to laugh about. He can choose whether he will be sad or cheerful. The change will not come easily or overnight, but with constant effort he can in time achieve something like the spirit of the woman who had to leave her home and her husband in the Far East when the war broke out there. She was pregnant at the time and subject to nausea. She was also susceptible to seasickness, and with two small children to look after, she had reasonable cause to feel thoroughly miserable, physically and mentally.

But since she couldn't better the situation, she chose to laugh at it. Sitting down to her first meal on board the ship, she noticed that three of her tablemates were also pregnant. So, reaching for the menu, she said gaily, "Well, let's see what we can find that will taste good coming up."

The neurotic who tends to the gloomy, self-pitying view might take to heart what one hospital patient learned about the business of getting well. Sure that he was very ill, much more so than he had been told, he tried the most devious ways to get evidence to support his discouraging conviction. One day when the orderly came in, he said to him, "Those second-floor patients are in pretty good shape, aren't they?"

"Pretty good, yeah," the orderly replied.

"There are some real sick ones on this floor, though, aren't there?"

"A few, maybe."

"I guess they put all the worst cases on this floor, don't they?"

The orderly looked at him a minute. Then he said, "You don't need a doc. All you need is somebody to tell you what not to think about."

Keep him occupied. Idleness at home is no better than in the hospital. There could be no worse treatment for the discouraged, despondent neurotic than to give him long idle hours in which to brood over his memories, his fears, and his weaknesses. There is no better treatment than to keep his hands and his brain busy with some occupation that makes him feel needed and useful again. A good job as soon as he is able to work, which in most cases will be right away, is the best possible medicine.

Remember, though, that the tense, nervous person must learn to balance the responsibilities of his job with recreation. All work and no play makes the neurotic not only a dull boy but a sick one. Good times with good friends he must have, but you may have to arrange them against his wishes for a while. He may feel sure that his friends won't want him around now, that they'll look down on him. Telling him differently won't do any good; his friends will have to show him by the warm welcome they give him, and by their continued friendship.

Give him a chance. Practically all these men will be able sooner or later to resume their former positions in the home and in the community, provided the family, the neighbors, and employers give them a chance. But if the mother takes over her son's life for him, stifling his initiative and his urge to get well, explaining to all comers that "Joe has to be careful now that the war's got his nerves"; if the wife is fearful, lacking confidence in her husband's ability to head his household again; if the employer hires him with the attitude that "the first sign of not measuring up and out you go"—then the man's chances for recovery will be poor.

The final goal of re-establishing the psychoneurotic veteran in the full life of the community is the job not only of his family, employer, and friends, but of every community organization: church, civic, professional, business, labor, or veterans'. In face-to-face natural contact these groups must be prepared to make the veteran feel at home again, not stigmatized or penalized because his injury or illness is of the nerves and mind rather than of the body. They must welcome him back for his abilities and potential contribution to the common cause. All he needs is a chance. They must see that he gets it.

SUGGESTIONS FOR READING

BARTON, BETSEY. *And Now to Live Again.* New York: Appleton-Century Company. 1944.

A good account of the feelings of a permanently disabled person and of the attitudes most helpful to readjustment, by an author who had herself to learn how to live again.

CHEVIGNY, HECTOR. "My New Eyes." *Survey Midmonthly* (September) and *Reader's Digest* (November) 1944.

The story of one man's experience in achieving new independence at Seeing Eye.

CLUNK, JOSEPH F. *Open Letter to My Newly Blinded Friend.* U. S. Office of Education. For sale by the Superintendent of Documents, U.S. Government Printing Office, Washington, D.C. Price 10 cents.

A primer of personal adjustment for newly blinded persons.

DAVENPORT, LT. MARSHALL. "Now I Can Go Home." *Saturday Evening Post,* February 17 and 24, 1945.

Two articles in which the author, a returned soldier, tells how he has fought his hardest battle against the silence, stares, and thoughtlessness of his countrymen.

FINK, DAVID HAROLD. *Release from Nervous Tension.* New York: Simon and Schuster. 1943.

A simple and clear description of the author's method of healing nervous tension — written in the hope that the book "will help the reader to find and inherit himself."

FOSDICK, HARRY EMERSON. *On Being a Real Person.* New York: Harper and Brothers. 1943.

A presentation of some important principles of mental hygiene by a minister who has had years of experience in personal counseling. It offers sound and helpful advice for those whose lives are complicated by nervous and emotional difficulties.

FURNAS, J. C. "Meet Ed Savickas." *Ladies' Home Journal,* February, 1945.

The story of a victim of combat fatigue, whose chances for complete recovery give hope to similar cases and whose wise handling by Mrs. Savickas can well serve as a pattern for other wives.

"Give Us a Break," by a returned flier. *Woman's Home Companion* (October) and *Reader's Digest* (November) 1944.

A man discharged for psychoneurosis recounts his experiences with family, friends, and employers.

MCGONEGAL, CHARLES C. "How I Get Along Without Hands." *Saturday Evening Post,* November 25, 1944.

NEUSCHUTZ, LOUISE M. *How to Help Your Hearing*. New York: Harper and Brothers. 1940.

PRATT, GEORGE K. *Soldier to Civilian*. New York: Whittlesey House. 1944.
A psychiatrist's description of the problems involved in the transition from military to civilian life.

Psychology for the Returned Serviceman. A Penguin book published by the Infantry Journal, 1115 Seventeenth Street N.W., Washington, D.C.
Written for the veteran himself, this little book, which sells for twenty-five cents, can also contribute to the family's understanding.

PUTNAM, TRACY J. *Convulsive Seizures: A Manual for Patients, Their Families and Friends*. Philadelphia: Lippincott. 1943.
A discussion and explanation of epilepsy for laymen.

RENNIE, THOMAS A. C., and LUTHER E. WOODWARD. *When He Comes Back* and *If He Comes Back Nervous*. National Committee for Mental Hygiene, Division on Rehabilitation, 525 East 68th Street, New York 21.
Two talks to the families of returning servicemen published together in a pamphlet that sells for fifteen cents.

STERN, EDITH M., with the collaboration of SAMUEL W. HAMILTON, M.D. *Mental Illness: A Guide for the Family*. The Commonwealth Fund, 41 East 57th Street, New York 22, New York. 1942.
In a simple and straightforward way this book, which sells for a dollar, discusses the problems to be faced by the family of one who is seriously ill mentally. The authors take the reader behind the scenes in mental hospitals and give specific directions for the family's guidance at each step from the onset of the symptoms to the reception of the patient back home after his discharge.

WALLER, WILLARD. *The Veteran Comes Back*. New York: Dryden Press. 1944.
A discussion of both the individual and the social aspects of the veteran's return.

WECTER, DIXON. *When Johnny Comes Marching Home*. Cambridge: Houghton Mifflin Company. 1944.
A history of how the United States has dealt with its veterans of previous wars. It emphasizes the need for jobs and for constructive handling of soldier attitudes.

YAHRAES, HERBERT. *Epilepsy — The Ghost is out of the Closet*. Public Affairs Pamphlet No. 98. Public Affairs Committee, Inc., 30 Rockefeller Plaza, New York 20, New York.
A brief discussion of epilepsy and epileptics that any layman could read with profit. It sells for ten cents a copy.

YOST, EDNA, in collaboration with DR. LILLIAN M. GILBRETH. *Normal Lives for the Disabled*. New York: Macmillan Company. 1944.
A book that will be of value to everyone who has a physical handicap of any kind. It gives a comprehensive picture of what has been and is being done to help disabled people rehabilitate themselves.

INDEX

www.ingramcontent.com/pod-product-compliance
Lightning Source LLC
LaVergne TN
LVHW052316200926
848481LV00002B/582